Praise for *THE* **SPARK**

*"I love that Chris cares so much about helping people. His honesty
and **The Spark**'s no-nonsense approach make taking control of your
life and achieving your weight management goals seem easy."*

— **Lisa Lillien,** *New York Times* best-selling author
and creator of the Hungry Girl brand

*"How do you ignite the spark to lose weight? How do you keep that spark
going so you can keep the weight off? This terrific book educates you and—
just as importantly—motivates you to eat and exercise in a healthy and
sane manner that you can keep up to become healthier, fitter, and thinner."*

— **Judith S. Beck, Ph.D.,** author of *The Beck Diet Solution:
Train Your Brain to Think Like a Thin Person*

"Chris Downie is Sparking a revolution of lifestyle transformation. **The Spark**
*is a royal win-win. The book lays down the blueprint for healthy living and the
Website provides an easy way for people everywhere to connect with likeminded folks.
Downie's passionate message is inspiring a growing, vibrant community of millions
of Americans to use their newfound health and fitness to achieve lifelong dreams."*

— **Pam Peeke, M.D., MPH, FACP,** Chief Medical Correspondent for the Discovery
Health Channel and author of *Fight Fat after Forty, Body for Life for Women,* and *Fit to Live*

*"**The Spark** strips away all the diet fads and baffling jargon to tell you what you really
need to know about getting healthy. With sound advice, simple plans, and jaw-dropping
before-and-after photos,* **The Spark** *will help you spark a revolution in your own life."*

— **Shauna Reid,** author of *The Amazing Adventures of DietGirl*

*"The SparkPeople program has had such great success because it's a
sustainable solution that works over time. There is great magic in this approach."*

— **Dave Ellis, RD, CSCS,** one of America's top sports nutrition experts; client teams
include winners of Super Bowls, the World Series, and college National Championships

*"Everyone has the opportunity to make a difference in the world. This book
is a great start to make a difference for yourself and everyone around you."*

— **Jeff Skoll,** founder & chairman of Participant Media and the
Skoll Foundation, and first full-time employee and former president of eBay

*"**The Spark** is more than just another 'diet book'—it provides a roadmap to a transformative health experience. It hits all the core elements of a healthy lifestyle and does so with energy, vigor and a true sense of optimism that comes through on every page."*

— **Martin Binks, Ph.D.,** clinical director & CEO, Binks Behavioral Health, assistant consulting professor at Duke University Medical Center, and author of *The Duke Diet*

*"This is an inspirational account of how one man started a dynamic movement which is helping people around the world fulfill a fundamental human longing—to achieve a healthy life within a supportive community of peers. More than a feel-good story, **The Spark** shows you how to harness positive thinking, implement sensible plans, and join a vibrant community. As a physician and researcher focusing on weight management, I'm thrilled to have this tool as a complement to the SparkPeople.com community."*

— **Kevin O Hwang, M.D., MPH,** assistant professor of internal medicine, research scientist, and weight management specialist at the University of Texas Medical School at Houston

THE
SPARK

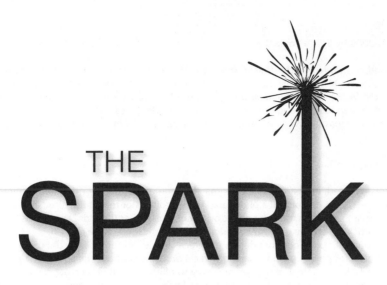

THE SPARK

The 28-Day Breakthrough Plan for Losing Weight, Getting Fit, and Transforming Your Life

CHRIS DOWNIE

(a.k.a. "SparkGuy")
Founder, CEO, and Motivation Expert
Along with the SparkPeople Experts and Members—
Over Five Million Strong

HAY HOUSE, INC.
Carlsbad, California • New York City
London • Sydney • Johannesburg
Vancouver • Hong Kong • New Delhi

Copyright © 2009 by SparkPeople, Inc.

Published and distributed in the United States by: Hay House, Inc.: www.hayhouse.com • *Published and distributed in Australia by:* Hay House Australia Pty. Ltd.: www.hayhouse.com.au • *Published and distributed in the United Kingdom by:* Hay House UK, Ltd.: www.hayhouse.co.uk • *Published and distributed in the Republic of South Africa by:* Hay House SA (Pty), Ltd.: www.hayhouse.co.za • *Distributed in Canada by:* Raincoast: www.raincoast.com • *Published in India by:* Hay House Publishers India: www.hayhouse.co.in

Design: Tricia Breidenthal

The author of this book does not dispense medical advice or prescribe the use of any technique as a form of treatment for physical, emotional, or medical problems without the advice of a physician, either directly or indirectly. The intent of the author is only to offer information of a general nature to help you in your quest for emotional and spiritual well-being. In the event you use any of the information in this book for yourself, which is your constitutional right, the author and the publisher assume no responsibility for your actions.

Library of Congress Cataloging-in-Publication Data

Downie, Chris.
  The spark : the 28-day breakthrough plan for losing weight, getting fit, and transforming your life / Chris Downie. -- 1st ed.
       p. cm.
  Includes bibliographical references and index.
  ISBN 978-1-4019-2645-8 (hardcover : alk. paper) 1. Weight loss. 2. Physical fitness. 3. Health. I. Title.
  RM222.2.D678 2010
  613.2'5--dc22
                              2009037769

Hardcover ISBN: 978-1-4019-2645-8
Tradepaper ISBN: 978-1-4019-2646-5

12 11 10 09   4 3 2 1
1st edition, December 2009

Printed in the United States of America

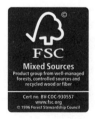

For the millions of people turning SparkPeople into a grassroots movement by reaching goals, helping others reach goals, and spreading the spark to more people. I hope this book does justice in bringing alive your passion and enthusiasm for making life an adventure!

CONTENTS

INTRODUCTION

The Spark Promise: More Than a Diet

A revolution is taking place—a community movement of millions of people discovering a new way of living and thinking about their weight, their health, and their lives. They are embarking on a journey with a proven system that builds confidence, supports personal growth, and inspires weight loss. And they are reaping great benefits, such as higher levels of happiness, more energy, improved health, the desire and ability to reach new goals, and increased connections with other people.

The old method of punitive dieting simply does not work. Complicated fads, rigid protocols, and a focus on deprivation lead to failure, as millions of yo-yo dieters can attest. But at SparkPeople the revolution is building. People are living better lives, making healthy choices, feeling great, losing weight, and keeping it off.

And their numbers are growing at an astounding rate. Every month, over four million people visit the SparkPeople Websites. And they are so passionate about their experiences that they are spreading the word, recommending the program to friends and family. In fact, 175,000 new members join SparkPeople each month—that's almost 6,000 per day, or 4 people every single minute of every single day.

The core of the program is an effective combination of nutrition and fitness with goal-setting techniques. But what makes this system so potent is the infusion of our own special magic—elements of a secret formula that make it accessible and profound as well as fun and rewarding. Our program radiates a joyous team spirit and the knowledge that people are nourished by each other as much as by food. We have created a system that promotes the interconnectedness of an extended family—mutual support and a sense of belonging that is healthy for both body and spirit.

To understand why SparkPeople is so effective, and why *The Spark* will have the same powerful impact, just take a look at the animal kingdom. Elephant trainers tether a baby elephant by a thick rope to a stake hammered into the ground in order to limit his range. Whenever the elephant tries to escape, he is quickly restrained by the bond, and he learns that he does not have the strength to break away. As the baby matures, the trainers reinforce the boundary set by this rope. By the time the elephant is an adult, he is massive, weighing several tons and capable of enormous feats of strength. But now the trainer could tether him by a slender thread and he still would not try to escape. The elephant has grown so accustomed to being restrained that he has no idea of the strength he possesses to free himself.

All of us are conditioned to live within a limited perception of our own power to transform our lives—moving through our days with invisible tethers that hold us back from becoming who we really are. But while the elephant submits to its restricted boundaries, we possess the freedom to set the scope of our own dreams. We're free to move out of the dusty circle where we've stood, stuck and discouraged, and into a new terrain that offers a landscape of vast potential.

We can awaken that smoldering spark inside ourselves and become our best and truest selves. I know because I have done it myself and so have millions of others.

WHY SPARK, WHY NOW?

There is a positive force that flows through you that is unique. At SparkPeople, we help you tap into it to envision your best life and then achieve it.

Take the time to do this now, wherever you are.

Focus on the core of strength and promise that resides within you, underneath whatever chaos your life may be in or whatever shape your body.

Give yourself up to this moment. Dare to see it.

Now look down at your feet; slip out of those invisible tethers.

Then ask: Where would you take yourself right this moment if you walked toward your most heartfelt dream?

What would your life look like? What would your body look and feel like? What level of energy would you have?

What might be your favorite activity? What would your daily life include?

Imagine happiness—the sweet glow of inner contentment, the way it tastes and smells and feels.

It may feel odd, even uncomfortable at first. As adults, we have grown unaccustomed to dreaming. We believe it's the domain of children or fools, of birthday cakes and wishing wells.

But our brains respond to wishing. Envisioning our hopes provides a path, as luminous as a beam of moonlight. Once you've visualized what you wish, an inner road is being cobbled for you to follow. Maybe you see yourself on a Hawaiian beach, slim and active. Or maybe you envision something more specific, like our member who dreamed of becoming a police officer, but was so heavy he had trouble getting off of his couch. A hundred pounds lighter after joining SparkPeople, he recently passed the agility exam for the Bakersfield, California, police department.

Or maybe, like our member Linda, you wish for increased mobility and health:

> *I am the lowest weight I have been in nine years, and I am proud of the fact that I did it from a wheelchair. I have lost over 50 pounds with my limitations. I was born with a disability and needed spinal surgery. I lost the use of my legs through the surgery and had given up. I ballooned up to over 300 pounds . . . I was homebound because of the wheelchair and had no access to a wheelchair van. I found SparkPeople, and it changed my whole outlook on life. I saw there was hope for me to be healthier.*

Although many people first come to SparkPeople for weight loss, our program is actually a way of life. A state of mind. It is a road map that will take you to a destination all your own: a place where you have confidence in who you are and what you can become.

As founder and CEO of SparkPeople, I've watched millions of others "spark" their lives to not only lose a tremendous amount of weight and achieve levels of fitness they never thought possible, but reach astonishing life goals as well—from healthier kids and family to improved career and financial well-being.

Our program inspires an inner power that not only connects you with others but also makes you capable of performing feats beyond your dreams.

Take Dana, a 45-year-old mother of three and grandmother of two who proves the far-reaching power of our program in a post she wrote on her online SparkPage:

> *Last November I was driving behind a bus doing the speed limit when from out of nowhere a car whips around both me and the bus. Yes, double yellow lines, on a hill, going around a blind curve . . . I freaked out and said to my son, "Oh my gosh, that person has a death wish!"*
>
> *After that corner the road becomes an upward progression of hills and valleys, so there's no seeing what's ahead until you're actually there.*
>
> *Sure enough, when we arrived there, it was a mess, a nightmare!*
>
> *I pulled over as quickly as I could and called 911. The car was in a ditch on the opposite side of the road about 50 yards from the car it had just hit head-on. Inside was a lady, probably in her early 50s; an airbag had punched her in the gut and chest pretty hard and she couldn't breathe. I was concerned she was having a heart attack because of the way she was grasping her chest. She was very much in shock and because of the enormous amount of smoke pouring in through the vents she thought the car was going to blow up, but there was no getting her out, so I got as much of myself as I could in through the busted-out window and held her.*

Finally, after several minutes, when the paramedics arrived, I had to let go of her and get out of the way, but I have to say, it broke my heart to let go, I didn't want to. This lady and I had bonded . . . and during those terrifying moments I had lost all sense of myself . . . there was no "ME" in the picture, only us . . .

The reason I'm telling this story is because all of you beautiful Spark-People cause me to have that same feeling, the feeling that I'm a part of something so much bigger than myself . . . That it's just as important to me that all of you become healthy and happy as it is that I do.

We live in such a busy, isolated society, there is so much loneliness and sorrow . . . so much stress and need of THINGS . . . when I was in that car with that woman, every bit of that vanished . . . all I felt was a desperate need for her to live.

I want you all to LIVE in every aspect of the word . . . I don't need to know you (although I'd love to) or be your close friend to know that you are a part of me . . . that the healthier you are, the healthier I am . . . that the more success and goals you reach, the more likely I am to do the same.

These are the kinds of stories I hear every day.

My own journey of self-discovery led me to SparkPeople. And thanks to the Internet, the Spark message has spread to millions of people—many of whose lives have been changed. But this book can do even more, connecting the dots between diet, fitness, community, confidence, and feeling good. *The Spark* delivers on the promise that dieting can be transformative. Its visionary system of support, motivation, diet, and fitness has a proven track record: nearly 10 million pounds lost and thousands of personal goals reached—and still counting.

SECRETS OF SUCCESS SURVEY

We recently sent a 64-question survey to a random sample of our millions of active members and received over 5,500 responses. The survey reinforces our program's core belief that the old, punitive dieting model is both outdated and ineffective.

This survey's compelling findings include dozens of practical ways to get results. We segmented the respondents into groups: people who reached their weight-loss goals, people who lost 100 pounds or more, people who called themselves "dieters," people who described themselves as "pursuing a healthy lifestyle," and people who reported being "stuck." The secrets of the most successful—those who either had met their goals or had lost 100 pounds and were on track to reach their final goals—are found throughout the rest of the book. You will learn:

- How our members have lost between 2 and 200 pounds—or more

- How so many of our members have gone from being winded walking to the mailbox to learning to jog, even run marathons

- How the majority of our members report increased levels of confidence, energy, health, fitness, happiness, and goal achievement

But perhaps the most striking result of our survey was the answer to this question: "If you are trying to lose weight or maintain your weight loss, which of the following best describes your efforts: *I am on a diet* or *I am following a healthy lifestyle*?"

Fully 90 percent of all SparkPeople members stated they were following a healthy lifestyle rather than dieting. Moreover, those on diets were much less likely to have reached their weight-loss goals than those living healthy lifestyles. People "on a diet" simply *lost less weight.*

Dieters tended to use tools that were centered on deprivation and willpower and focused on the scale. Healthy lifestyle members, on the other hand, used strategies that were focused on positives, eating more fruits and vegetables, cooking *more* healthy foods, eating substantial, healthy breakfasts, and drinking much *more* water. They had a major philosophical difference from dieters who viewed their plates as half empty, while they viewed their plates half full.

The old diet model that you need to grit your teeth and suffer is not only antiquated, it doesn't work. This is the crux of why our members finally achieve lasting weight loss, improved fitness, and better health as well as greater levels of personal happiness.

WHAT YOU SHOULD KNOW ABOUT SPARKPEOPLE

SparkPeople has become a veritable village green of motivation and participation where your journey becomes energized by the powerful support and community of other people who are "sparking their lives"—both online and offline. Members regularly e-mail, talk, and get together; they inspire, encourage, and challenge one another, and even hold one another accountable. Throughout the book, you'll meet many of our members and hear how joining the SparkPeople community has changed their lives. You'll see them mentioned by their SparkPeople username, which is how they are identified on the site and to their friends in the online community.

In a recent poll of our members, the majority of respondents reported a dramatic increase in happiness after joining SparkPeople. A full 30 percent went from reporting the lowest level of happiness (1 on a scale of 1 to 5, 1 being least happy and 5 being happiest) to near the highest (a 4 or 5). And fully 90 percent of *all* respondents reported that they were somewhere at the top of the happiness scale.

The SparkPeople team includes health and technology experts who are passionate about helping people reach their goals. Our community consists of millions of people who help us continually improve the program and Website so we can keep helping more people. And our members give us motivation by reaching their big goals and shouting out on our message boards, "If I can do this, please believe me that you can too."

But this book is really about *you*. Your goals and dreams. What's most important to you? What goals would you like to start reaching today? What life do you really want to live? It's all possible when you learn the secret formula for the Spark.

The Spark is a completely different way of thinking about diet, fitness, reaching your goals, and living your life. Where most diets are compartmentalized programs separate from the rest of your life, with many rules and restrictions, the Spark is about your whole life. It's about what you *can* do, not what you *can't* do. It's about celebrating and building on your victories and learning from your missteps, not about focusing on a quick fix that so often leads to a "quick ditch." It's an innovative way of discovering that losing weight is not an end in itself, but rather a means to an end. The larger rewards of losing weight and being fit are:

- Gaining confidence by setting and reaching small goals
- Building, nurturing, and belonging to a community
- Gaining inspiration, encouragement, and connection
- Igniting passion, fire, and an adventurous spirit
- Sharing the spark with others—and seeing it grow
- Living a better, brighter, bigger life

If you've never heard of SparkPeople before, or if you don't spend time online, this book will deliver everything you need to discover this new way of thinking and to put it into practice. If you are already a SparkPeople member, this book provides a simple yet powerful 28-day program that, for the first time, distills the most beneficial aspects of SparkPeople into an accessible, easy-to-follow format. Even if you've been involved in a healthy lifestyle for some time, this 4-week program can be a great way to refresh or jumpstart your efforts. And as you go, if you ever need a "fallback" program to restart your momentum, this will work well for that, too. No matter where you are, this is a great way to return to the basics of what really works, build a strong foundation, and sustain your momentum so you can get the most out of your new lifestyle

This book will also deepen your connection to the program, providing for the first time the history and framework that are at its foundation, as well as exciting new content—including a deeper exploration of our philosophy. And *The Spark* will give you a more portable and tangible source of ongoing inspiration, to place by your bedside or take along on your daily commute. This will dramatically increase your chances to reach your most important goals.

THE SPARKPEOPLE MAGIC FORMULA

We've distilled the best of a medically accepted, common-sense nutrition and fitness program and infused it with our own magic in order to make it accessible, profound, and far-reaching in its scope and effectiveness.

Our secret formula combines such innovative elements as:

- *Goal-setting:* A system of visualizing your larger goals that gives more meaning to your daily actions, and a way to create and build confidence and momentum that fuels results

- *Behavior change:* Using wisdom from the science of behavior change to help you turn the tide on negative behaviors and effectively replace those unhealthy habits with healthy ones that then become a natural, even enjoyable, part of your life

- *Community support:* Inspiring real-life stories of ordinary people who've transformed their lives, and a 24/7 source of help and encouragement

- *Positive motivation:* Points, trophies, and awards that transform dieting into a fun and exciting adventure

- *Team building:* Affiliations with other members based on geography, hobbies, interests, and amount of weight to lose

- *Accessibility:* A program that easily fits into the most hectic life, building momentum while remaining entertaining and fun

- *World-class technology:* Tools, content, and community, continuously updated, often from suggestions by SparkPeople members

The core of the book and the underlying philosophy of the SparkPeople lifestyle is an innovative program of personal empowerment. It includes four cornerstones that make up the building blocks of living a "sparked" life:

1. *Focus* is the ability to set priorities, live a life according to your values, and become clear about your vision and goals.

2. *Fitness* is a physical and mental springboard that provides you the energy to reach your goals and trains you to think on your feet.

3. *Fire* is the passion that is created by your actions and momentum. When you live with fire, you see possibilities, not problems.

4. *Positive force* is what happens when you share your energy and success with others. The more you give, the more you get in return.

The second component, the four-stage SparkDiet, is a customizable, step-by-step journey that offers the tools, confidence, and motivation to jump from simple dieting to a healthy way of life so you can reach not only your weight-loss goals but much more.

An important element that makes the Spark authentically different from other diets is that it includes the positive community support that can be the key to sticking with any program. Changing your life in a vacuum can be very lonely; human beings are communal creatures who need each other. Like the SparkPeople Website community, this book will offer a method for creating community and connection online, offline, or both.

And, perhaps best of all, the program is fun. It is built on a system of positive rewards in which people can earn points for every positive step they take toward a healthier lifestyle. And it is imbued with a sense of playfulness and adventure that our members tell us they've never before found in a weight-loss program. We believe strongly in making health and fitness fun—how else can we be expected to make and stick with healthy changes? The Spark does not focus on punitive restrictions and rigid regiments. It is about what will really work in your life, and how you can maintain these healthy changes and live with a sense of adventure and happiness.

THE SPARK PROMISE: SPARKPEOPLE UNITE

I know the Spark program works because it has been carved directly from my life. But if I couldn't spread the word to others, it wouldn't be the success it is today. The stories of SparkPeople are nothing short of inspirational.

Take Ann, the wife of a sailor stationed in Japan.

When you're a woman who weighs nearly 280 pounds, a look at your goal weight on the charts can be an exercise in humiliation. The extra weight seems so enormous that the notion of losing it via the usual methods—the airy diets in women's magazines, stressing grapefruit and carrot sticks—feels nearly impossible. These plans seem to be designed for someone other than you—someone with a different character or life. They don't take into account the truth of your experience, the way people treat you as if your weight is a flaw reflective of your character, how the simplest social outing can be an occasion for the deepest self-consciousness—a trip to the beach in a vast, skirted swimsuit, the derisive look of a waitress when you order chocolate cake for dessert.

Then there are your doctor's warnings of how you're putting yourself at risk of type 2 diabetes, arthritis, and cardiovascular problems. Not that you need anyone to tell you this, because you already feel it—your knees hurt when you stand too long, and your heart pounds when you run up a flight of stairs after your child. You've tried other diet programs with their humiliating weigh-ins and punitive calorie tallies, where you end up eating your quota by noon. These programs seem drenched in deprivation and leave you feeling alienated and alone.

You only have to try and pick up a bag of mulch to realize how heavy 50 pounds is and become discouraged all over again that you have this—and more—to shed.

It becomes easier to isolate yourself and open another bag of potato chips, to dream vaguely of gastric bypass surgeries or other miraculous interventions. It's easier to feel disillusioned, stuck, and ashamed. Being a serviceman's wife is stressful enough, moving from one base to another, acclimating to another culture, making new friends. But living in Japan, a slender society where even clothes are sized smaller, weighing over 250 pounds can make you feel like a giant.

The Japanese live by the maxim *hara hachibunme,* eat only until you're 80 percent full—a practice from Okinawa, which may have the longest life expectancy in the world. But Okinawans live longer not just because they eat well, but because their culture also places a premium on community, meaningful activity, fitness, and engagement. Okinawans work throughout their lives, passing on their skills and providing encouragement to younger members of their society.

These components are also part of the SparkPeople program and are essential to its success compared with other diet programs, which have a dismal success rate.

Ann's journey illustrates why our program is so successful. After a friend invited her to join, she thought about the core reasons why she wanted to lose weight in the first place—in order to preserve her health, to feel good about herself again, and to provide her son with a strong role model. She broke down her goals into what we call "streaks"— small, sustained activities that she committed to performing regularly—beginning with short aerobic workouts. She became aware of how and what she was eating, made small substitutions in her diet—mustard for mayonnaise, mineral water instead of soda—and added fruits, vegetables, and whole grains. She began to track her fitness activities and daily calories on our online tracker. These moves weren't drastic, but they were regular and powerful. Ann met new friends online who faced the same challenges, who shared their stories and congratulated her on her successes. Visiting message boards, she realized that her own experience could be an inspiration, and she eventually became a program motivator herself.

The benefits of the program spread throughout her life. When she went on vacation, she spent time exercising with her son. She didn't sabotage herself by trying to follow a drastic diet, centering on no carbs or no fats, but instead ate a gently modified version of what she really liked. When she went shopping, she rewarded herself with a beautiful dress that she would have been unable to button six months before. And her SparkPeople friends were always there, a click away, on her laptop.

She was able to do all this because the Spark plan was a pleasurable lifestyle that she had incorporated into her life through incremental steps over time. She had constructed a firm foundation, not the kind of sand castle her son built on the beach, which was swept away by the first strong wave.

Ann discovered the powerful satisfaction that arises when you change your own life. So far she has lost over 80 pounds—and gained so much more.

MY START

When I first started SparkPeople I had a simple goal: I wanted to help millions of people. To anyone who knew the shy, quiet boy I once was, this might have sounded like a ludicrous proposition. I may now live in a house near Silicon Valley with a view of the Pacific and a wife and two young sons who are my chief motivation for staying healthy and goal-oriented.

But it wasn't always like this for me.

CHAPTER 1

MY STORY

I think of the past as a region, and I can still see myself there: it's 1980, and I'm a scrawny kid with a latchkey dangling from a crocheted loop around my neck.

I was an awkward child, so painfully shy that the only way I could deal with people was to march by them with my head down, my gaze pinned to the ground. Books were my escape and comfort. I opened them and fell into a world of adventure.

I lived with my mother and younger brother in Cincinnati, Ohio, in a time and place in which successful boys possessed brute strength and an easy confidence. That wasn't me. I was the skinny little kid, shorter than average, and nicknamed Rubber Band, because I got knocked down so often when I went up against the big kids in soccer games yet always bounced back.

My father had exited our lives for the most part when I was six, and it had been left to my mother to raise my brother and me. I could tell it wasn't easy. In fact, my mother and I seemed to share some general unease with the world that I didn't have a name for yet.

We had moved significantly downhill since my parents' divorce, leaving our house for an apartment complex replete with thugs and petty criminals whom I spent much of my energy outmaneuvering. My brother and I had to pare down our possessions and even give up our beloved dog. We lived from paycheck to paycheck.

A passionate gardener, my mother now had only a tiny flower patch and a small patio to greet her once she opened the front door—but she kept her dreams alive with that small plot. That she'd had to give up perennial borders, along with so much else, made something ache inside me.

I'll buy you another house one day, I silently vowed, watching as she began her second shift of the day, cooking and cleaning for my brother and me. On the face of it, such musings were laughable, given that I was so timid that I couldn't even bear the sound of my own voice. Yet in spite of my shy exterior, another person was secretly lodged inside me—a budding entrepreneur who was ambitious, courageous, and full of promise.

That was the real me, a successful leader who would someday emerge and break free from this bashful prison, though I wasn't sure how this would ever occur.

As it was, I had an overwhelming fear of drawing attention to myself. Talking—one-on-one or in groups—was terrifying, and there were whole days when I spoke to no one except my family. But the one thing that trumped my nervousness was a desire to do well in school. Somehow I managed to raise my hand in class and achieve good grades.

Soccer, which I gradually become involved in, also helped; I had an early realization that exercise made me feel not only stronger but also less nervous. It also forced me to become part of a team, working toward a common goal.

By high school I gathered the courage to mention in class that my goal was to become an entrepreneur, though no one knew what that was. So I sat back and fed my secret self with books and daydreams.

Thanks to student loans and a job at a refrigerator-magnet factory, I headed to the University of Cincinnati—a mini-city of 30,000 students—after graduation. I was excited to take business classes, though dismayed by the gigantic campus. I continued living at home, punching a time clock at 6:00 A.M. at the magnet factory, and working a shift before heading to classes.

I majored in accounting because numbers were still easier for me than people. Much of my academic performance was due to intense cramming. I had a good memory and stuffed it full of data, then disgorged it at the designated time. This got me A's, but I wasn't learning much as I was packing my brain with facts that later exited my mind entirely.

One of my requirements was a public-speaking course, an activity that topped my list of terrors. In my first speech I set out to explain how to make my mother's secret chili recipe, but for all my nervousness you would have thought I was explaining the theory of quantum mechanics.

I'd brought the ingredients and set them up at a table, but my hands were shaking so hard that I kept knocking things over, including tomato sauce, which dripped off of the desk like blood. My lips trembled, and my face was covered with a sheen of sweat as I blurted out the steps: "Sauté the onions, then add the beans!" I felt like I might faint right there, in front of my classmates. I got a D minus for my efforts, but only because the professor obviously felt sorry for me.

For someone who was accustomed to A's, this felt like a calamity, and I redoubled my efforts. The rest of my speeches were so highly memorized that it was as if a robot were delivering them. I eventually got an A in the course, but I knew I still had a problem.

By then, I had begun to see that what my mother and I shared was something called anxiety, a term that hardly seemed to cover the vast disquiet that overlay our lives. My anxiety made me increasingly competitive; I became committed to overcoming it, which I did in a haphazard fashion.

I challenged myself by taking another public-speaking class on a pass/fail basis. I made a rule that I wasn't allowed to overprepare or memorize my speeches.

Even more importantly, I cut myself a break—a breakthrough for me. I told myself that I was allowed to make mistakes without beating myself up. This not only gave me the freedom to try new things but also it helped me with another realization. When you suffer from anxiety, you feel as if your faults and flaws are so apparent that everyone is watching you, assessing all that is amiss. But I gradually realized that people didn't care as much as I thought about my every move. This was liberating, and it made this class one of the best moves I'd made.

In the second half of college, I joined a low-key business fraternity and began some cautious socializing, which led to more involvement in fitness and athletics. I saw again how exercise produced overlapping effects—reducing my anxiety as it gave me energy and increased my confidence. I also interacted with people, although initially this wasn't the case. When I first began my fitness program, I was still mostly alone at home, working on a cheap weight set in my bedroom and doing hundreds of sit-ups and push-ups.

I also did repetitive sprints up and down our driveway, barreling down the blacktop, then coming to a screeching halt at the street. Of course, drivers didn't realize what I was doing and often swerved and honked when they saw me coming.

Still, it was yo-yo fitness. Great spurts of overworking combined with a total decline once school became too hectic—the same thing, I realized later, that happened with people who repeatedly dieted.

ONE SPARK CAN LIGHT A LIFE

Once I graduated from college, I landed work at Procter & Gamble as a staff accountant. My job was to roll up accounting numbers for seven factories and share them with financial forecasters.

P&G was known for hiring young people straight out of college, and then throwing balls in the air to see how many they could juggle before they began to falter. Being such an overachiever, I didn't want to drop a single one, and I was soon juggling as fast as I could.

It was a great job and P&G is known as one of the top companies in America to work for, but I quickly got sucked into the wrong way to "make it" in corporate America. My fitness had come to a halt—there was no time for it now. I rushed to fast-food drive-thrus at lunch and sat in the car, wolfing down oily fries and meat patties dripping with cheese. I knew this was emotional eating, but I didn't care. This respite was sometimes my only pleasure in a stressed-out day. By the time I got home in the evening I felt as if I had been cored with a knife. I collapsed on the couch and absorbed whatever flickered in front of me on the television. I felt as if my energy and stamina were leaking out of me, like a deflating balloon. From the outside, I was performing well, but this was hardly the future I had envisioned for myself.

A co-worker down the hall, a lumbering, heavyset man twice my age, often stopped by my cubicle. "Well, I've got eight years, seven months, and six days until I retire," he said one day as he left. I watched him walk down the hall and felt a dreadful bond. The perks, the salary, the stress—I knew how easily I could morph into this man in a decade or two.

I realized there had to be a better way to fulfill my life. During lunch breaks I began reading goal-setting and leadership books, speckling the pages with ketchup. For the first time I made myself seriously focus on what I wanted for my future—to specifically name and visualize it.

Why did it feel so odd, even embarrassing, to actually write down what I wanted from my life? Why hadn't I ever done this before? Some of my goals surprised even me. It turned out I definitely wanted a family of my own, something I hadn't quite articulated before. I wanted to be healthy and eventually become a successful entrepreneur with my own business. I wanted to make money and do positive things with it. Little did I know that the early design for SparkPeople was beginning to take shape.

Next I went through magazines and put together a vision collage—photographs that represented these goals. These photos may have looked like typical action photos of healthy-looking people playing sports with friends, but embedded in them were my secret desires, which I'd never told anyone—not even, until recently, myself. Several photos symbolized leadership and business success, along with a reminder of a goal that I had set for myself—that I'd leave corporate America after two years unless I was happy.

I pinned the collage to my office wall and looked up at these images when I was adding columns of numbers, fielding urgent deadlines, and feeling discouraged. They made me remember what I was working toward. Each choice I made every day gave me the chance to get one step closer to my goals.

A STREAK OF LIGHTNING

I decided the best way to motivate myself was to combine goal-setting and motivation with fitness, a crucial link in my self-improvement plan. I began what I called a streak, a sustained period of positive activity—ten minutes of daily exercise each morning.

Even this wasn't easy. One icy morning when I had to get up at 5:00 A.M. for a monthly closing, my charming, lazy self said, "Come on, Chris. It's too early—you don't have to work out today." But then my dedicated side challenged, "Come on, you've done this for 34 days in a row—you don't want to break your streak."

Looking back, I see that this streak and the positive self-talk were two tools out of many that I used to become accountable to myself. This was a big change. Prior to this, I would often silently blame others when something went wrong. Now I realized that I needed—and wanted—to be responsible for my own actions. It was powerful to learn that no matter what happened to me, I could choose how to respond. And so with my eyes still half closed, I got down on the floor and began doing sit-ups. Within a few minutes, my fatigue had passed and I'd woken myself up, in more ways than one. My blood pumped and my thinking cleared. There were my goals—I could see them again.

These small workouts—only ten minutes out of a 24-hour day—paid immediate premiums, providing me an inner momentum and energy. Even though work owned me for 60 hours a week, I began to feel that I had a grip on my own destiny.

My performance at P&G improved significantly, and I won a promotion. I made attempts to improve my windowless cubicle, bringing in a light box and potted plants and playing classical music on the radio. I realized that I was finally figuring out the "right" way to thrive in corporate America—or to meet any other challenge in life, from career to parenthood—and that anyone could do this.

The positive effects began crossing over into other areas of my life. My morning workout made me more energetic and positive throughout the day. Now I was more likely to take a walk at lunch instead of sitting in my car, gorging alone on greasy food. I was more likely to have the energy to stop at the gym on the way home from work.

I found myself interacting more easily with people, actually deriving pleasure from conversation. For the first time ever, I was astonished to realize that I rarely felt shy and anxious anymore. I remember driving down the road one cold afternoon and actually having the most foreign thought: *I feel happy.* It wasn't just the "normal" type of happiness I had felt many times before, like everyone else. This was different, a kind of exuberance, as if I were filled with some inner fire, as if I could do anything.

At first, I didn't mention my streak to anyone else, but as the days added up, I began to talk about my workouts when I was on the job.

A co-worker of mine named Pat had an office right across the hall from me that was decorated with decades of photo milestones. She was 20 years my senior and probably 50 pounds overweight. She had an ironic yet affectionate manner with me, as if I were her slightly addled son.

"So Chris has worked out 50 days in a row, and I've sat on the couch for 50 days in a row," she announced one morning in the lunchroom to general laughter. She said this as a joke, but there was a certain resignation in her voice that touched me. It wasn't that she was miserable, but she seemed stuck—in this job, in this body, as if there was nothing that could ever change it.

Then one morning, when I was nearing the 100th day of my streak, I was standing in my doorway when I saw something out of the corner of my eye. I turned and saw Pat hanging up a sticky note on her own door—with the number 1.

"I worked out this morning," she said proudly, then walked to her desk and sat down. Her ironic tone had vanished.

All that day I found excuses to leave my desk and look at that note on her door. By the end of the day it was seared in my mind.

Not long after, Pat was transferred to another location in Cincinnati, and we stayed in touch via e-mail, probably once a week. When she wrote that she was having difficulty keeping up her daily workout, I encouraged her to persevere. I realized that encouraging her was helping me stay on track.

I had now done over 200 days and had become a veritable powerhouse of energy. I'd never helped around the house before, but now instead of going home and lying on the couch after work, I began doing dishes and vacuuming, dashing around at a frantic pace.

"What's gotten into you?" my mother asked.

"I don't know—I've just got so much energy!"

I could tell she was grateful for the help but a little bewildered all the same.

When I got into work one day, six months later, a co-worker said to me, "Have you seen Pat?"

"No, why?"

"She's here for a meeting. You won't believe it when you see her."

He was right, I didn't. When she walked into my office later, it was as if a slimmer, brighter version had emerged. It wasn't simply the weight—though she'd lost a lot of it—it was a new energy and freshness, a lightness in her step.

She began telling me in an animated tone about the walking club she'd established at her new location, and how many other women had joined it because they saw the changes in her. They had told her, "Pat, if you can do it, we can do it!"

Then she said, "Chris, I want you to know you changed my life."

I couldn't believe the effect these words had on me—the jolt of exhilaration and surprise, as if I'd been brushed with a live electrical wire.

The final component of my self-improvement program finally clicked into place. That spark, that component of sharing and connection, was what had been missing.

The notion that I had helped this woman—by encouraging her, involving her in my goals, and being a positive role model—was one of the most startling and gratifying realizations of my life. Of course, I said none of this to Pat as she stood there in my office. My shy alter ego may have begun fading, but he was still there, huddled inside; I was so overcome by Pat's words that I had to avert my gaze, afraid I might cry.

She must have realized this because she made an excuse to leave, but in her wake a new thought hung in the air: *Your daily actions and words impact more people than you ever realize.*

I had started this adventure working to reach my goals. But now that I'd motivated Pat and she'd motivated a whole group of others, I began to consider how many people everyone together had touched—and what they had accomplished from this motivation and what they might accomplish in the future.

I took this encounter as a sign and put together a short outline of my improvement plan and began showing it to others. This was it—what I had been vaguely searching for! Now I was determined to somehow turn this into a business that helped many people.

Pat made me realize that weight was the area where most people become stuck and disillusioned. As they gained pounds, they lost energy and confidence; they didn't feel like exercising or eating anything but empty comfort food; they isolated themselves and grew discouraged. It was a cycle that I knew could be broken and redirected.

I didn't have a weight problem myself, but I'd spent enough years sitting on the sidelines, eating alone in my car, and lying on the couch in listless exhaustion, to know it was all related.

Thus the Spark program was born.

FROM EBAY TO SPARKPEOPLE

As I continued working on my program, I began meeting with Rob, a college friend, who was also restless in his corporate job. We decided to leave our jobs to co-found a Website, Up4Sale.com, where people could bid for products online.

After about a year, Rob and I brought on two additional partners—Tom and Wally— and an intern named Josh to lead much of our technology. We rented the attic of a dilapidated mansion near downtown Cincinnati for $500 per month.

Those two years of building our small company were the hardest of my life. At 26, I experienced my first taste of bootstrap entrepreneurship. I was so poor that when the lease on my car ran out, I couldn't afford to renew it, so a friend gave me a 13-year-old, ramshackle Toyota. One window wouldn't go up and another wouldn't go down. During one winter ice storm, I found myself scraping the insides of windows coated with ice as I drove along the deserted freeway at three in the morning (yes, you read that right!). Needless to say, I had no personal life.

We kept expenses low, going so far as unscrewing light bulbs from fixtures with multiple sockets to save money. Even so, I ended up putting $50,000 on my own credit cards, which I paid off with other credit cards. It was a dangerous game that could come crashing down in personal bankruptcy if the company faltered—which, on many occasions, seemed likely.

By 1998, I was working 100 hours a week, rarely leaving my computer screen because of all the activity on our site, staying awake until 3:30 A.M. every night to monitor it. We were growing so rapidly, that we caught the attention of eBay, whose competitive-intelligence team had been keeping an eye on little Up4Sale.

Later that year, they flew us to their San Jose offices and offered to buy our company for eBay stock and enough cash to pay off my credit cards. We also had a salary for the first time in years.

When eBay held its IPO, we had the bizarre experience of watching our stock explode in value before our eyes. What had started out at $14 a share grew within the year to $800 a share—nearly $100 million divided between our four partners—before a large contribution to Uncle Sam, of course.

My Toyota, as if registering my new fortune, bit the dust—the brakes failed as I was driving to work one day, and I had to veer off onto the side of the road. Finally, I allowed myself to buy a new car. I moved out of my mother's house and rented an apartment.

In October of 1998, eBay hosted an off-site party in California to celebrate the IPO. I didn't want to go because it was on my birthday, but a top executive wanted me to represent the Cincinnati office.

At the party, held in a beautiful wooded retreat near the Pacific, I met another eBay worker, named Karina, who was the liaison between eBay and top sellers.

When I told her how I hadn't wanted to attend because of my birthday, she said, "That's funny. I didn't want to come either. It's my birthday too."

Hmmm. Interesting, and so was she, I thought, regarding her out of the corner of my eye. I had a few drinks, so perhaps that explains why I was agreeable enough when one of the executives paired me with Karina and insisted we slow-dance together in front of the gathering as the "birthday couple."

This was a potential powder keg of anxiety for me, but I felt oddly calm. It wasn't simply the drinks. After a lifetime of feeling out of place, awkward, and tongue-tied, I felt amazingly comfortable in this young woman's arms.

Maybe my body registered what my head still didn't—that this was the person I could finally be myself with, who would love me and join together with me to form a central part of my secret vision collage. Right beside my dream to be a successful entrepreneur, I also deeply desired the kind of safe and stable family that I hadn't known in my own childhood.

The lights twinkled and the ocean roared; in Karina's hair I caught a lovely scent that I later recognized when I held our newborn sons. But that was the future, and I learned in that long dance to savor the astounding and miraculous present.

STRIKING OUT ON MY OWN

A year after the IPO, I began selling my eBay stock; I was suddenly worth more than I could have imagined. Some people have difficulty figuring out what to do after sudden wealth, but not me. As soon as I caught up on my sleep, I turned back to SparkPeople, the personal-improvement program that I had wanted to use to help others all along. The name "SparkPeople" comes from our mission to "spark" millions of people to meet their goals.

My mother watched as I made these moves. She saw the tangible results one afternoon in 2001 when I drove her through a leafy suburb and pulled up in front of a house with perennial borders and flowering shrubs.

"Who lives here?" she asked. "I was thinking maybe you would," I replied.

She looked over at the flower beds and then back at me; the expression on her face was enough.

That was a big couple of years for me; I bought the house for her, and Karina and I married, after several years of long-distance courtship.

I was still deeply lodged in my hometown, so Karina joined me in Cincinnati, though I could tell it was difficult for her. She wasn't accustomed to "real" winters. Later I joked that I had won the battle but not the war.

I finally decided it was time to break away from eBay and strike out on my own; I wanted to start something that had the potential to change the world. I used the profits from my stock sales as seed money to start SparkPeople and hired several employees to join me in setting up a Website.

The final pieces of the puzzle were falling into place. The basic principles of the SparkPeople program had helped me reach personal and professional goals beyond my wildest dreams. I had learned from Pat that other people could use the same principles to reach their goals.

During those first five years, I put up $5 million of my own money to finance the development and salaries of an amazing team dedicated to helping people. This was a significant investment for me, one that has impacted a number of my life decisions.

Karina was a great support, and she followed a modified version of the SparkPeople program herself when she became pregnant, along with another early SparkPeople employee named Rachel. This resulted in such easy, healthy pregnancies for them both that their doctors asked them, point blank, "What are you doing?" We realized that there were no Websites at the time that focused on healthy pregnancy, so we started one called BabyFit.com.

My wife wasn't the only one transformed by her pregnancy. I had never been a kid person before—that is, until we had William, our first son, and then our second, Nicholas. Then it was as if a wind had blown through and altered me completely. I was a father now, a role that I had had little experience with growing up, and this made me committed to doing the best I could as a dad. I was amazed to see the boys copy my interest in exercise.

Cincinnati was hardly a hotbed of Internet activity; it became clear I couldn't personally fund our business indefinitely and that we'd eventually need funding, likely from Silicon Valley. Karina, who had cooled her heels in Cincinnati for over four years, finally won the "war," and we moved to the West Coast.

In 2006, we decided to make the SparkPeople site free for anyone to join so that we could help many more people reach their goals. Our site grew more and more popular—to become, according to comScore, the most active diet and fitness Website in America. Just as I'd hoped, we received funding—from Steve Case, co-founder of AOL. Steve was passionate about improving health care and thought SparkPeople could grow into something special.

This was the first real move of my life to a place that was so different from my upbringing. I was the same guy in many ways—I still showed up to work in a SparkPeople T-shirt and shorts—but inside there was a major difference. I had achieved so many of the goals that had been embodied on the glossy magazine pages I'd hung on my wall at P&G. But it still felt like there was unfinished business—that the most important part of the adventure was ahead of me.

Sometimes when I walked into a room of our house near San Jose, I regarded my new life with dazed gratitude and disbelief. There were my wife and two tawny-haired sons bent over a book—there was a view of the ocean in the distance, a blue shimmer still dazzling to my landlocked Midwestern eyes. This scene was especially poignant for someone like me, who grew up thinking he needed no one but himself, who believed he might just end up spending his life alone.

That's why I don't mind keeping the shy boy I once was tucked in a corner of my mind—he's an active reminder that personal transformation happens everyday to ordinary people like me.

He's also an active reminder of how far you can climb when you spark your life's goals with focus, dedication, and the connection with others.

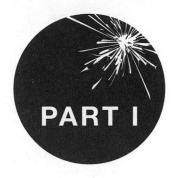

PART I

THE FUEL FOR IMPROVEMENT SYSTEM

The Fuel for Improvement System is the philosophy behind the successful Spark-People program. It is powered by four cornerstones—Focus, Fitness, Fire, and Positive Force—with each cornerstone containing several building blocks. Traditionally, people have treated these topics—especially fitness—as stand-alone, isolated areas for improvement. What they don't realize is that these four areas of life work together (or against each other) to determine how "sparked" their lives can become. My goal in developing this philosophy was to bring together all the areas that can help people improve and reach their goals. I especially wanted to show how different areas of life are more connected than we realize.

Our philosophy is individualized. You can start in any cornerstone, with any building block, depending on your initial goals. As you improve in one area, your actions cross over and build upon other areas at the same time—what we call the "crisscross effect."

So don't be surprised if you begin to see positive changes and your life improving in ways you never expected. Taking steps—both large and small—to stoke each of these areas begins to fundamentally change how you think, how you act, the kind of life you're living, even the person you are.

Everyone knows that exercise and nutrition are intertwined. But have you ever considered exercise and leadership? Or goal-setting and sleep? Each building block and cornerstone is directly linked with all others. Each has a powerful potential to act as a foundation that naturally sparks other areas as progress is made. And the short-term goals you select as part of your program can have a positive impact on several areas at once. Improvement may come from a completely unexpected place. To reduce stress, you can use traditional relaxation techniques. Or you can tackle the problem from a different angle by starting in the Sleep or Nutrition building blocks. This means you can tailor your pursuit of results to fit your needs and interests.

TANGO5617, a member, uses the image of scaffolding to explain how this worked in her own life:

> *I've lost nearly 40 pounds so far . . . then I maintained that weight loss through about seven different life stressors (ended an engagement, quit a job, moved, death in family, serious family illness, moved again, started new job). Looking at my life now, I see that I've changed in so many ways. None of it happened overnight; it all happened one choice at a time. Scaffolding really works—the idea that you can take success in one area and use it to build success in other areas as well. For example, my newfound awareness of nutrition in the grocery store has led to a greater awareness of cost, which led to better budgeting. Learning how to break down huge goals such as "lose weight" has helped me begin to break down another huge goal, keep a clean house—it all ties together! So, on my second anniversary of SparkPeople, my habits are healthier, and I've learned to succeed. I'm lighter in body, stronger, and more able to tackle everyday challenges. I'm happier and more able to choose my happiness. I'm even a nicer person.*

Like TANGO5617, you might also discover that improvements in one area of your life lead to a natural desire to improve in others, especially when you take advantage of our motivational techniques. One of our favorites is a system called SparkPoints, a way of making all types of goals enjoyable and fun. We use it on our Website, and we've also built a SparkPoints motivational program into this book so that you can earn points and even win prizes—including a motivational phone call from me—on your journey to weight loss and a healthy, successful life. To learn more and start earning SparkPoints now for reading this book and taking the steps it suggests, go to Appendix E.

As you continue reading this book, you might encounter an idea or technique and find yourself thinking, *That won't ever work for me.* Just keep in mind that as you take small steps along your journey, techniques that may not have worked for you in the past might start being successful as you weave different areas of your life together in a new, exciting way.

For example, we hear all the time from members who can't believe how they have come to *love* exercise and eating healthy foods. The idea is to add elements to your life that are fresh, interesting, and fun—no matter where you start—knowing they'll impact other areas.

We use this philosophy as the foundation for the specific steps and program in Part II. As you read, try to consider how each cornerstone and building block might apply to your goals. By having this big picture in mind, you will be far ahead of most people trying to reach their goals—and you might end up using your successes to motivate others, as so many other SparkPeople members do!

CHAPTER 2

CORNERSTONE:
FOCUS

Imagine you suddenly found yourself adrift in the ocean with a life preserver but no idea where the shoreline was. As far as the eye can see, there's only the same wide blue vastness. What would you do? Probably tread water, battling waves and struggling against the current. But without a clear direction you'd soon grow discouraged.

That's what life is like when we have no focus. We drift about—going to work, paying our bills, reacting to whatever comes our way, but feeling rudderless. We may even be happy for the most part. But eventually days turn into years and we find ourselves so far off course that we've lost track of the dreams we once had.

Having focus provides a reference point, a lighthouse on the horizon to swim toward with enthusiasm and hope. It prevents us from floating, adrift in our own personal sea. To make any lasting change or achieve any meaningful goal, you need to know where you want to go and how you're going to get there.

Without a goal line, the game of football makes no sense, and neither does the game of life.

The day I sat down in my windowless cubicle at P&G and actually made myself focus on what was important to me was a turning point.

Before this, my life was a hectic blur, a rush from one disconnected activity to another. I gobbled my fast food meals; I met deadlines; I made occasional sprints up and down my driveway. But I was really headed nowhere.

Like most people, my typical day was choked by dozens of situations where I was tossed about by external events. A phone call, a complaint, a co-worker's action might derail any vague plan of my own. My future seemed to be spinning out ahead of me of its own accord. I saw myself, as if in a time-lapse photograph, sitting in the same chair as my hair grayed and my body bent. It wasn't that being an accountant in a large corporation was a dreadful future; it just didn't feel like my future.

Like most people, I'd been vague about my goals—as if I somehow didn't deserve to have, let alone attain, them. I carried around a knapsack of half-baked wishes, ideas of what I *should* want, and comparisons with others. In this way I drifted around like a cork in the ocean, letting the waves of external events and other people's expectations define my destination.

Yet one of the surprising discoveries of positive psychology, a field that focuses on what causes happiness, is that contentment and meaning in life do not arise from the usual suspects—winning the lottery or being young and beautiful—but, among other things, through the pursuit and attainment of goals.

That day when I finally focused, I wrote that I wanted to eventually:

- Have a strong family and relationships
- Become an entrepreneur
- Learn how to overcome my shyness and anxiety
- Be healthy and fit

Initially it felt a little odd, almost selfish, to focus so intensely on my personal desires. During all my years in school, I had never learned the first thing about focus or goal-setting. I had been taught subjects such as woodworking, geometric theorems, and how to convert inches into centimeters. Yet no one had mentioned this nearly magical skill—one of the most essential of all. Once I thought about what was most important to me in life, I started turning those thoughts into goals.

I had grown used to squandering my hours as if they were *Monopoly* money, but concentrating on my real focus changed all that. I began noting the activities in my day that were distractions. What was the point of the two hours I spent languishing in front of the TV, talking aimlessly on the phone, complaining about my job?

Now instead I took mini-vacations where I soaked my mind in the positive images hanging over my desk. I might have been a young accountant working on difficult deadlines, but in my mind I basked in the glow of love and friendship and the power of being a successful leader.

These small but potent steps illuminated a path for me to follow and gave me a pleasurable sense of direction and purpose. I realized that focus had been missing from my previous attempts at self-improvement and fitness—disjointed, chaotic efforts without cohesion. But after that fateful day, I wasn't just aimlessly sprinting down my driveway anymore. Even if no one else could see it, I was running somewhere specific now—to a future I would live down the road.

The power of focus became clear when a local insurance adjuster named Calvin visited the SparkPeople office one day and told our team, "I need to lose weight."

He said this in the reflexive, downbeat way that people often speak of weight loss—as a burden, another thing they should do. When we asked him why he wanted to lose the weight, he shrugged, as if he'd never actually considered this before.

"I just need to," he said.

As we spoke with him longer, Calvin began talking about sports and grew animated about a recent basketball tournament. When he took out his wallet to find a schedule, there was photo of a boy with a buzz haircut and a smile identical to his. Calvin looked down at him and his face softened.

"He's the reason I want to lose weight," he said after a moment. "I want to be healthy so I can play basketball with my son."

It was easy to see that Calvin deeply valued his family and that one of his main goals in life was to be a great father. We encouraged him to write this down and build a vision collage. Then we helped him break down his goal into small action steps. Sure enough, when we saw him several months later, he had lost the 20 pounds because he had his real goal in mind.

Focus often arrives after an "aha moment"—an event or emotion so powerful that we're stopped in our tracks and say: "Wait a minute. Is this how I really plan to spend the rest of my life?"

That happened to member Elizabeth after she underwent a mortifying experience.

> *I decided to change my habits when I was kicked off a carnival ride for exceeding the weight limit. It was humiliating but eye-opening. I found SparkPeople and tracked everything religiously. I joined a gym and loved group classes so much that it inspired me to learn to be an aerobics instructor. Setting mini-goals has been the greatest tool I've used, and the support of the online community has been indispensable. I went from couch potato to fitness enthusiast, lost 80 pounds, and made some of the best friends I've ever had.*

Erin's focus was her daughter.

> *After the birth of my daughter I hit an all-time high in my weight—255 pounds while pregnant and 225 pounds one year later. One day my husband and I sat down and decided we needed to do something. We didn't want our daughter to grow up heavy and learn an unhealthy lifestyle. Our daughter was our wakeup call.*
>
> *A friend of mine found the SparkPeople Website and sent it to me. By making small changes I started to notice small changes. The site encouraged me to start exercising more, so I began to run. The weight started to come off more consistently. The weight loss, along with my family, kept me motivated. Over the last year I have lost over 90 pounds.*

GOALS: DREAMS WITH DEADLINES

The Japanese carp, or koi, has the ability to grow according to the size of its environment. Placed in a small tank, it grows to no more than two to four inches, but if placed in a larger body of water, it can increase to three times that size.

Luckily, humans don't physically expand and contract based on the dimensions of their surroundings. But we do develop emotionally, intellectually, and spiritually according to our environment. While the carp has no choice but to accept the boundaries of its world, we are free to overcome our limits and chart the dimensions of our lives.

That's where goals come in—setting them is at the heart of the SparkPeople program. The habit of focusing on goals provides the essential framework for all parts of your life, the blueprint for your deepest desires. Most importantly, goals bring meaning to everything you do. When you're leading a life geared toward a mission, even the most mundane tasks seem to take on significance. Rather than dreading them, you face them with new energy and dedication.

The SparkPeople program encourages members to focus not only on long-term goals but also on smaller intermediate goals and action steps. Long-term goals are usually one year or more, but can be shorter depending on the goal. Medium-term milestones are usually one to three months. Short-term action steps are usually less than one month.

In my case, once I had focused on what I desired, I set two long-term goals for myself. The first was to leave corporate America within two years to start my own company unless I found a way to be fulfilled and happy where I was. Second, I wanted to become fit and healthy over the next year.

Such long-term goals were essential because they acted as a game plan and gave me control over my life. But in order to build momentum, I knew I needed to start small and be consistent. So I broke my long-term goals down into two action steps:

1. A countdown of 730 days, which would motivate me

2. A "streak," a sustained positive activity that would get me started—in my case, ten minutes of fitness every day, usually in the morning

These daily and weekly goals kept me on track and allowed me to launch immediately on to the path to my new healthy future. Completing them gave me continuous satisfaction and motivation that fueled my journey. Importantly, everything I did fit easily into my normal daily lifestyle. I wanted to build a plan that I could stick to and keep making progress.

My medium-term milestone, which I initiated later, was to focus on each 100 days of my fitness streak as a grouping and to initiate regular meetings with my friend Rob to bolster my focus and brainstorm. This three-month period was short enough to focus on achieving important results that contributed to the long-term goal. Talking with Rob kept my long-term goal fresh and alive; sharing my ideas kept me enthusiastic about performing my action steps. Bridging the gap between short and long term with medium-term milestones can make your journey more pleasurable and keep your "fire" burning.

For me, the crisscross effect from this laddering of goals produced beneficial effects across all areas of life—my long-term focus and daily exercise began to reduce my shyness, give me energy, and increase my confidence so I was more comfortable interacting with others. Each day had purpose.

BUILDING BLOCK: VALUES AND BELIEFS

We all have a deep wish, an inner inkling of what we want to accomplish and the values we want to live by. But with so many distractions, it's often hard to hold on to—like a golden cord that is pulled further away as the years go by.

To be powerful, your goals should be aligned with your core beliefs and values. When you are clear about your values and beliefs, they are a natural part of your daily actions. Each goal and decision is rooted in them, like flowers in soil. And these values act as both an anchor to keep you grounded in what you believe and a compass that helps guide you through your adventure.

But what if you haven't truly figured out your values and beliefs yet? That's fine. This is something so important that we don't expect you to figure them out in a few minutes. Simply keep them in mind and come back to this section later after you have had more experience in other areas.

Think about:

- What truly drives you?

- Is there a clash between what you really believe and what you're trying to accomplish?

- Are you working each day toward something that really matters to you?

For example, having a strong work ethic and the desire to provide for your family might be a deeply held value that helps determine your purpose in one or more roles.

I always knew I wanted to be a successful entrepreneur, but I had no idea when I started at P&G that helping other people would become so essential to my life. It wasn't until later, when I saw how my own actions had inspired my co-worker Pat, that I became aware of a burning desire to help others.

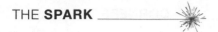

Linking my desire for success with this other deep impulse really put me on track. But I couldn't have arrived at this realization without first following my initial process of setting goals. The benefits of my program crisscrossed and enriched each other, sparking new realizations and unexpected growth.

BUILDING BLOCK: PURPOSE AND VISION

Locating your purpose and your deepest life intentions can help you move with greater clarity each day of your life. Your purpose is what defines your life. It's more than your occupation or daily responsibilities; it's the reason behind your existence. Being a great mother or making a positive contribution to your community may be your purpose. You can even have a purpose for each role in your life—as an employee, a parent, a spouse, or a community member.

Your purpose is drawn directly from your values and beliefs as water is drawn from a well. Your purpose then becomes the foundation for setting your goals.

Your vision is what your future looks like when your purpose becomes a reality. There are tools to help you envision this future, using the strength of your powerful mind.

There's a fable about a prisoner sentenced to a life of punitive labor—all day long he turned the crank of a machine that provided light for a nearby town. It was monotonous, tedious work. But when he gazed out of his small prison window he could see lights on the horizon. He was exhausted each evening, but he took pride in the fact that he'd spent his day in a useful enterprise.

After years of work, another inmate told him: "You're not creating light—that's from the electric generator across town. When you turn that crank all you're doing is pushing paddles through sand in a drum. You're just wasting your time."

The prisoner investigated and found out that this was true—his turning the crank was completely unrelated to the production of light. When he had felt his work had meaning and purpose, he was able to deal with any setback and survive his ordeal. But once his illusion was burst—once he saw his work was useless—he grew despondent and lost hope.

As the philosopher Nietzsche once said, "He who has a why to live can bear almost any how."

BUILDING BLOCK: GOAL-SETTING

We all need to feel that our goals are infused with purpose. One of our members, Laura, a divorced mother and businesswoman, was desperate to lose weight but had been unable to find a method that worked for her. As a sales rep for a printing company, she traveled during the week, ate on the run, and often snacked in the evening in her hotel room, where she found herself exhausted and lonely for her children.

When she joined SparkPeople, we asked her to take the time to focus on her real purpose and values. When she did, she discovered the clash in her life that had stymied her weight loss and had left her so discouraged.

Her values and core beliefs were centered on being a responsible person who lived with integrity, and her main purpose was to be a good parent. But since her divorce, she had been faced with the challenge of making enough money to support her family. With her current job, her mother took care of her two small children while she was on the road. This created an inner conflict that left Laura depressed and fueled the eating binges that had caused her to gain over 50 pounds.

What she really desired was to work locally so that she could spend more time with her family and be a fit and attentive breadwinner and mother. She had buried this wish because she knew how much her family needed her income, and she didn't believe there was any way she could find comparable work closer to home.

She is an example of how we often short-circuit goals before we even set them. We listen to the hectoring internal voice that says: *You can't have that. Who do you think you are?*

It also illustrates how weight is often the symptom of deeper issues—in Laura's case, a problem with the very way she was living her life. The extra weight she carried was an added burden that made her too inert and depressed to initiate a new job search.

Your body is the vessel in which you live out your life. Living in a body that is stressed, unfit, and overweight impedes your journey. We encouraged Laura to focus on exactly what she wanted and to write it down.

She wrote: "Within a year, I want to lose 40 pounds and find a local job so I can be a fit and attentive mother and breadwinner."

Laura's statement reflects the essentials of good goal-setting. Goals should be:

- *Unique:* A goal shouldn't be something that your wife wants for you or part of your office mate's New Year's resolution. To be effective, it must be all yours. It must arise from your deepest personal desires and passions.

- *Concrete:* Goals should be exact and time-specific. "I want to be fit some-day" or "I want to lose weight" is too vague. You should try to define your goals in concrete, tangible language. "I want to lose five pounds in four weeks" is a realistic, concrete goal that can be measured and tracked. How-ever, since it's often tricky to set specific weight-loss goals for a variety of reasons, you should be flexible with this one.

- *Inner-directed:* Losing weight or becoming fit because you're feeling dissatisfied or you're comparing yourself with a slender model isn't a positive goal because it is outwardly focused rather than coming from inside you. Losing pounds for your reasons will make your journey unique and powerful. You won't be trying to fit into anyone's clothes but your own.

- *Harmonious:* Your goal shouldn't conflict with either your values and beliefs or your life's purpose. If you want to be a wealthy businessperson but believe deep down that making money is immoral, the clash between your goal and your deep beliefs will inhibit your progress.

- *Realistic:* It probably took you years to gain the 20 pounds you want to lose, and you can't possibly lose it all in a week—without going into starvation mode. But you can lose one or two pounds in that time. Start off with a goal that is challenging without being so overwhelmingly ambitious that you lose sight of it. Then remember to break it down into small, gradual steps.

- *Written:* There's something powerful about the act of writing down your goals. They are no longer ethereal thoughts or wishful thinking, but there on the page in black and white. That's why we ask you to explicitly spell out your main objective, being as tangible and specific as you can. You'll be amazed at how this kind of concrete focus clears the way for you to begin moving in the right direction. It brings you out of the fog, where it is difficult to navigate, into the sunshine where your path is clear.

Break Them Down

Once Laura came up with what she really desired, we encouraged her to break her goal down into long-, medium-, and short-term components.

Her *long-term goals* were to find a job closer to home and to lose 50 pounds to be healthier for herself and her family. Her *medium-term milestone* health goal was losing the first 10–20 pounds. Her *short-term action steps* for this goal were to take a 15-minute walk every evening and to drink eight cups of water per day.

One thing you'll learn is that long-term goals often overlap with each other. So, in this case, working on her health goal helped Laura build confidence and contributed significantly to her job goal.

By breaking down her goal into these components, she was able to take immediate small steps that kick-started her gradual weight loss, increased her focus, and gave her hope and energy. Acknowledging small victories gave her confidence that she was on the right path.

It's important to choose a few high-priority areas that are motivating and in line with your values. Pay attention to those until you form good habits in these areas. Then move on to the next. The idea is to find the sweet spot, that special place where different goals converge and support each other.

The confidence and accomplishment that arise from a steady stream of progress are great motivators. Setting and reaching a string of goals, no matter how small, is a regular dose of satisfaction that will one day bloom into pure inspiration.

Seeing It

Seeing your own purpose and goals, actually envisioning them with intense focus and concentration, is a kind of visualization, a powerful technique that has been used by peak performers.

Charles Garfield, a doctor who has done research on such top performers, studied NASA astronauts and observed how they repeatedly rehearsed in simulated environments the actions they would eventually perform in space. He found that peak performers, whether in sports or business, were visualizers who trained their minds as well as their bodies. They developed powerful mental images, seeing in their mind's eye their ultimate goals and the steps to achieving them.[1]

Imagery is the language our brains use to communicate. The average person forms at least 50,000 thoughts and images every day, many of them negative. Most of us are quite adept at concentrating on negative thoughts and imagery, such as *I'll never lose this weight* or *I'm going to be stuck in this job forever.* But with a little practice, you can use your imagination in a positive way by envisioning your desired goal.

Take a few moments several times daily to envision yourself, as vividly and clearly as possible, living your best life—doing what you wish, alongside the people you love, in a setting you desire. There you are, slender and fit, jogging down a sunny beach with your children. There you are standing in front of the mirror, smiling at the reflection of yourself, healthy and strong. There you are performing the small, daily steps that will lead to your goal—driving past the fast-food drive-thru, exercising ten minutes a day, sitting down with your friends to a healthy meal.

See it, experience how it feels, and visualize your own best potential.

In this way, you are creating an inner movie that you can tune in to whenever you wish—in the middle of a traffic jam, while waiting in line at the bank—whenever you have a moment that could be wasted with stress or worry.

This is a technique that is available not just to CEOs and gold-medal winners, but to all of us—a powerful way to channel your energies toward your own unique goal.

Saying It

The words we say, internally and externally, have tremendous power, yet they're often full of doubt and fear. Converting your goals into positive statements or affirmations is another way to focus intensely.

Replacing negative inner dialogue with upbeat thoughts floods the mind with positive messages. Simply saying aloud each morning and evening that you are going to achieve the things you want is a potent way to remain focused.

Scott Adams of *Dilbert* fame tells of how he wrote 15 times a day the affirmation: "I, Scott Adams, will become a syndicated cartoonist." Ten years later, that's exactly what he'd become.

Writing what you wish 15 times a day may seem excessive, but think of how many times each day you tell yourself "No" or "I can't."[2]

Affirmations that can be tailored to your life include: "I am happy, healthy, and free," "I possess health, wealth, and love," and "I am willing to spend the energy and time to make my lifestyle healthy and happy."

I can vouch for the power of affirmations from personal experience; I've used them for years, especially this one: "SparkPeople will succeed and help millions of people." In fact, my sitting here writing this book today is the result of countless repetitions of this affirmation.

Positive affirmations also promote optimism, another component of a meaningful life. People who are optimists expect positive things and are more adept at noticing and taking advantage of opportunities around them. And optimists tend to be physically and mentally healthier and better than pessimists in overcoming negative experiences.

Affirmations also promote gratitude—taking time in the middle of life to savor one's blessings. Another contention of positive psychology is that people who give thanks for their good fortune rather than dwelling on their misfortunes are generally healthier and happier. Rather than happiness making them grateful, it seems that being grateful helps create their happiness.

NOW, YOU

Aristotle once said that man is, by nature, a goal-seeking animal whose life only has meaning if he is working toward a goal.

I found the most inspiring example of the power of goals in Viktor Frankl's book *Man's Search for Meaning*. Frankl chronicles his experience as a prisoner in a concentration camp during World War II. He explains that while others died of illness or simply gave up living, his motivation to survive was his simple goal to write a book about his new form of psychotherapy.

I remember sitting at the picnic table in my mother's backyard in Cincinnati reading the words of this old survivor from another time and country. Then I came upon a passage that grabbed my heart.

> *We who lived in concentration camps can remember the men who walked through the huts comforting others, giving away their last piece of bread. They may have been few in number, but they offer sufficient proof that everything can be taken from a man but one thing: the last of the human freedoms—to choose one's attitude in any given set of circumstances, to choose one's own way.*[3]

I put down the book and looked around me. It was a balmy spring day in Ohio, and I was a healthy young man living a free life in a time and place where I could follow any dream that I wished. I could stand up at this moment, climb into my car, and drive wherever I pleased—south toward Florida or north toward Canada. I could say whatever I wanted and pursue any goal.

If Frankl could manage to hold on to his dreams in the midst of such unimaginable suffering, surely I would be able to overcome my own small challenges and find a way to persevere with my life's goals.

So can you. No matter who you are, you have the key within yourself to live your own best life by simply channeling your vast potential and energy toward a goal that encompasses your own unique vision and purpose.

Start now by asking yourself:

- What are your core values and beliefs?

- How can you turn those values and beliefs into a purpose in one or more of your life roles?

- Visualize your purpose. How can you see it becoming a reality, based on where you are now?

Later, we'll ask you to be more specific about writing down these goals and then breaking them down into short-term, medium-term, and long-term goals. But for now, let these questions roll around in your mind, and see where they take you. And remember, there's a simple test to help determine whether your mission on earth is completed yet: if you are alive, it isn't.

CHAPTER 3

CORNERSTONE:
FITNESS

What if I said that you could begin transforming your life by simply walking back and forth to your mailbox every day?

Maybe you'd laugh or tell me I was crazy. Yet we've had members who could barely get out of bed or bend to tie their shoes who ended up running marathons and losing over 100 pounds by starting out in just this way. From under the rubble of old pounds, they were able to recover the fit and vital selves they had never expected to see again. Becoming reacquainted with the strong body and mind within you that function in harmony—moving, thinking, eating, and sleeping—is what we call *fitness.*

Take a moment and visualize the healthy, vibrant person who is living inside you. You may have left her—or him—sitting on the sidelines for years, but that doesn't mean she isn't ready to reemerge.

See that shining self in your future. She doesn't have to look like a movie star or a model—simply you, at your best. Keep this image in mind as you continue your Spark-People journey until that day when you look up and meet her, face to face, in the mirror.

That's what happened with our member Andy:

SparkPeople has transformed my life. I no longer look at food as comfort. Now I see it as fuel for my beautiful machine. I actually look at myself in the mirror! I love who I see. I have made many small steps to make lifelong changes to better myself. Everywhere I go people comment on how good I look, but I feel it from the inside so much more. I am confident and willing to try new foods, exercises, and even challenges in life. I look at each new day in a new light. I've probably added years to my life, and I am forever grateful for that. Clothes look better, shopping is fun, and even food tastes better! I am worth it. Now I can see.

THE BALANCE OF FITNESS

If our great-great-grandparents could see how we live, they'd probably be shocked by how sedentary modern life has become. Our forebears were accustomed to moving their bodies—tending fires, carting water, and walking wherever they needed to go.

We, on the other hand, can spend an entire day barely moving a limb—sitting at computers to work, to shop, and to exchange e-mails, cruising in cars for drive-thru meals, and reclining on couches at night. Yet movement is a central characteristic of human life; our bodies are made for locomotion. And like our tribal ancestors, we flourish when we take time to relax, share good food and companionship, and then revitalize ourselves with restful sleep.

One day when I was passing an acupuncture office, I saw a diagram of a human body composed of an intricate design of swirling, interconnected meridians. It was so colorful and arresting that I stopped for a moment and studied it. The diagram was so different from depictions of the body I'd seen in specialists' offices—a length of spine, a slice of skin, a model of a knee, as if each of these were separate entities, disconnected from the rest of the body. But this chart showed the body as a unified river, with many colorful tributaries flowing throughout. That's how we think of fitness at SparkPeople.

The Fitness cornerstone is also designed with a unified flow—with all parts of the body and mind linked together. Mental and physical fitness place you in an optimal position to focus and become clear about your goals. This "unified flow" concept also relates to the connection between the four cornerstones. Increased energy and stamina boost your ability to take action, building momentum and fire. And fire puts you in the position to be a positive force for others and the world.

The components of the Fitness cornerstone also have crisscrossing effects that build upon each other. Exercise is a proven stress releaser that may cause you to crave healthy foods, such as fruit and vegetables, as well as water.

Exercise often changes the personality of your body and mind; instead of pondering what kind of salty snack you want next, you might find yourself casting a yearning eye toward salads and smoothies, the very kind of nutrition that will continue to make sustained exercise and goal attainment possible.

In turn, exercise and optimum nutrition help you attain a good night's sleep. You'll be authentically tired from your exertions, not jazzed up on caffeine and sugar. And restful sleep will make you raring to go in the morning.

It's like a giant jigsaw puzzle, with each component clicking into place. Leave out a piece and you may miss part of the picture. Include them all and you can have the whole lovely landscape of promise and success.

BUILDING BLOCK: EXERCISE

Even as a child, I knew physical exercise held part of my salvation. From the age of six all the way through high school, I played soccer. The crisscrossing effects of this single activity were remarkable to me even then—with this one sport I was able to use both my brain and body, join with others to form a team, and work toward a goal. I may have missed some easy soccer goals because of my anxiety, but there were many moments of triumph.

Exercise Will Get You There

If exercise is such an amazing booster, why do so few of us find time to do it?

At SparkPeople, we hear three common reasons: "It takes too much time," "It's hard/painful/boring," or "I'm no athlete."

The truth about exercise is actually the opposite of these statements. Let's turn them around and see why SparkPeople members—ordinary people just like you—end up becoming so excited about exercise that they can't imagine not doing it because it makes them feel so great.

Exercise Makes Time

Yes, it sounds crazy, but exercise truly does give you more time instead of taking it. How is this possible?

Imagine yourself sitting in front of your computer all day. How do you look? You may be slumped in front of the keyboard, your back out of alignment, your neck stiff, your eyes focused on one spot as you perform repetitive movements that stress your wrists and hands. Sitting in a stationary position like this is exhausting, and after several hours, your productivity drops because of stress and fatigue. At SparkPeople we encourage our employees to get up throughout the day and take quick exercise breaks, even if for only a few minutes.

Our employees stretch, jog in place, roll their necks and wrists. They even close their office doors and do push-ups or jumping jacks, or they leave the office for a midday run outdoors or to hit the nearby gym. These quick breaks recharge both mind and body. We find that employees get more work done even though they've taken a few minutes off. And they feel revitalized, happier, and more productive. SparkPeople employees and members even report that they often get their best work ideas during exercise sessions!

Yet this is only the short-term picture. The astounding benefits that occur when you include exercise consistently for months and eventually years are threaded into the fabric

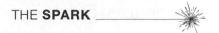

of your daily life. Such a regular and integrated fitness program will wake you up, build endurance, and provide energy and clarity to keep you moving toward your goals.

Make Exercise Easy

The words "exercise" and "easy" don't often go together. Most people think exercise needs to be hard, painful, and even punishing. In fact, the way most people design their exercise program, it *is* hard, painful, and punishing!

Here's an example of the typical way that people initiate an exercise program, the "I want it now" method. After reading and hearing from her friends how good exercise makes you feel, Susie says, "Hooray, I want to feel great, so I'm going to get in shape, and I'm going to get in shape right now!" Even though she hasn't exercised in years, she heads outside with the goal of running a mile.

The first minute or so, she's ecstatic, admiring her reflection in the windows she passes—she feels sleek as a gazelle and proud of her new resolve. *This will be a cinch,* she tells herself.

Yet it isn't. A distance that only takes a few minutes in a car seems to last forever. Suzie feels it in her knees and lungs; after three or four minutes she starts to lag and tries power walking. But soon even this is too hard. Her heart's pounding and she's covered in sweat. What had started out as a feeling of triumph and possibility sours as she walks the rest of the way home.

Oh, well, she thinks, *I guess I wasn't meant to be a runner—I'm a failure at yet another activity.* By the time she arrives home, she's abandoned her fledgling exercise program, which was alive for less than an hour.

In our quick-fix society, Suzie's error is a common one. Had she instead set a goal to jog—or even walk—a quarter-mile and done this successfully, everything would have been different. She would have reached a goal instead of "failing," and she would have been excited about the next goal.

Secret of Success: Don't Give Up!

Don't like to exercise? Take heart. Of those people in our Secrets of Success survey who met their goals, only half of them actually liked exercise before they started Spark-People, but a full 75 percent like it now (and a full 96 percent either like it, love it, or at least love how it makes them feel when they're done.) Of the dieters in our survey, on the other hand, 64.5 percent did not like exercise before and only 38 percent like it now.

THE EXERCISE TIPPING POINT

When you first begin an exercise program, you need to put a great deal of effort into it for what seems like small results and benefits. This doesn't seem fair. And it wouldn't be fair if the situation lasted forever. But it doesn't! When you make these efforts consistently and for a long enough period, you eventually reach a magical "tipping point." In his book on the topic, Malcolm Gladwell writes that such tipping points are "the levels at which the momentum for change becomes unstoppable . . . the moment of critical mass, the threshold, the boiling point."

Once you hit that point in exercise, the original equation reverses and you receive more results and benefits relative to the effort you put in. Your body slips into gear like a racing bike, and the ride becomes smooth, pleasurable, and productive. This tipping-point concept applies to many SparkPeople System building blocks but is easiest to see in action with exercise.

My own exercise tipping point came after three or four months, but it's different for everyone and has many variables, including the crisscross effects from other building blocks throughout the SparkPeople System. Take a look at the other building blocks in fitness, as well as those in the other cornerstones. If you aren't getting enough sleep, this will dramatically impact when and whether you reach your exercise tipping point. Same for nutrition: if you're living on cookies and soda, your body isn't receiving the proper fuel it needs to perform regular exercise.

We accept the tipping point without question when it comes to learning other new skills. Let's say you begin learning Spanish; during the first few months, you're not proficient enough to have a fluid conversation or read a book. But once you've mastered the language and use it consistently, it becomes part of your life. You don't have to start over every day boning up on grammar and punctuation. It's simply part of who you are.

Yet there's something about exercise that makes us feel that we should immediately be transformed and feel ecstatic. I believe this is the single most common reason why people never develop the consistent exercise program that could change their lives.

Consider it from your body's perspective. It has been accustomed to sitting around with its feet up. Now all at once you are asking parts of yourself that may have been dormant for years to move, flex, and bend.

"Whoa, what's going on here?" your body asks as you begin pushing it. "What are you asking me to do with these quads, these triceps, and these ankles?"

That is why SparkPeople emphasizes starting small, staying consistent, and building momentum. Begin your exercise program with any small and measurable fitness goal. It doesn't matter if it's as easy as walking down your gravel driveway every day. As I mentioned earlier, we have seen people use such simple actions as a springboard to losing 100 pounds.

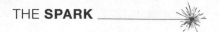

Once you reach your goal, you'll be so excited that you'll almost automatically want to know what's next. And by starting small you'll slowly signal your body that things are changing, giving it time to adapt instead of breaking down.

When the program "kicks in" you'll discover the jubilance and power of truly feeling fit. Here's Justin:

> *My journey began over five years ago. As I started the uphill battle against my body, all I understood was the pain and struggle it took to get through a workout. After a year, I began to notice some serious results. Along with my shrinking waistline, my mind was becoming sharper. What-ever the reasons, I was getting better in my studies and more assertive in my work. When I came home from university, my family and friends constantly commented on how I had changed physically. These positive affirmations meant quite a bit to me, but the most important words of encouragement were not "Wow, you look amazing!" but "Wow, you're a whole different person!" With a healthier mind and body, I realized how much of life I was missing when I was 280 pounds and fat and lazy. Now, after over five years of living a healthy, active lifestyle, I have lived dreams I never thought possible. I have completed adventure races, climbed mountains, walked on the Great Wall, and learned how to use my health to serve my community and the world. Now I am a United States Peace Corps volunteer working in Romania. There is no way I could have done that five years ago!*

Everyone Is an Athlete

We often hear people say, "Exercise isn't for me; I'm not an athlete." Unfortunately, these labels can be self-applied at a very young age and then stick for the rest of a per-son's life. If this applies to you, get ready to rip off the label!

The truth is that everyone is an athlete. We all have the right, privilege, and freedom to use our miraculous human bodies to their fullest potential. Sure, we can't all be Olym-pic swimmers like Dara Torres, or play soccer like Mia Hamm or basketball like Michael Jordan, but we can do our best. And then strive to do a little better the next time, just like our member Sara.

> *I personally started last summer and HATED working out. Now I find exercising very enjoyable and just signed up for my first triathlon! I never thought that was possible. I was the girl who couldn't run the mile in gym class, and the teacher just finally stopped timing. But with SparkPeople it*

has become fun. I look forward to working out, and it has become part of my day. I look forward to future challenges, and I now know that I can accomplish anything. ANYTHING! Why should athleticism be reserved for only an elite few? If I can make it this far, then you can too!

Here's an example from my own "athletic" career. At one point in my mid-20s, I read about the benefits of jumping rope in building endurance, coordination, and agility. So I bought a jump rope and started to jump in the basement or driveway whenever I had the chance.

I quickly discovered that it wasn't as easy as it looked. Jumping rope involves timing and coordination, neither of which I could immediately muster. I couldn't do more than five jumps in a row without tripping or stumbling. I knew I looked like the dorkiest person in the world. I felt like a failure, goofy and awkward. I'd seen schoolgirls jump double Dutch—managing two jump ropes that spun like egg beaters, even reciting rhymes. What was the matter with me?

The "old me" would have simply given up. But I challenged myself. I said, "Come on, Chris, set a goal to jump ten times without missing." I persevered and got to ten jumps. Then 25, 50, 100, 500, 1,000, and more. At some point, it just clicked, and I was elated to realize that I had reached a goal, that I had conquered this skill and was good at it.

That was 20 years ago, and jumping rope has been an essential part of my exercise program ever since. Because I started small and improved consistently, I can now jump rope insanely fast. It's so much fun, as well as being a great cardiovascular workout. I take my jump rope on business trips and have been known to jump rope in airports, on sidewalks in front of my hotel, and even in the hotel room if there's enough space (apologies to the people in the room below me).

I recently jumped in front of my hotel during a stay in Washington, D.C., and used it as an opportunity to "spread the spark" to a curious woman working at the front desk.

Make Exercise Part of Your Lifestyle

Another barrier in developing a consistent exercise program is life itself. It becomes really big, messy, and busy sometimes. Kids, work, exams, family—something is always right around the corner, ready to derail our best intentions.

When I was first developing the SparkPeople program and focusing on the link between fitness and goal-setting, one of my streaks was doing ten minutes of fitness at home with simple equipment. Going to the gym was icing on the cake—it wasn't a chore, because I already had the foundation of the small home workouts. As a result, I never had the excuse that I didn't have time or couldn't get to the gym. This ten-minute workout strategy was like magic for me because once I started, I usually went longer—and going longer felt like extra credit! Getting started is often the hardest part. But, on busy days, even doing only ten minutes meant that I had reached my goal and stayed consistent to build momentum.

I tried to convince my athletic brother, Joe, to try this philosophy, but he didn't buy into it. Instead, he went to the gym four to six times per week and got into really great shape over a brief six-month period. Then suddenly exam week came around—and he also had to continue working at his job. There simply wasn't enough time to go to the gym. So he fell off the wagon, a result of burnout and not having something simple in his program that was an easy jump start.

This was such a crucial moment. There's a law in physics that says a body at rest tends to stay at rest and a body in motion tends to stay in motion. This law also applies to our bodies.

Because the gym made up Joe's entire exercise life, he didn't engage in any fitness at all for nearly a month. When he decided to get back into shape, he had to start over nearly from the beginning. Those hundreds of hours he'd already invested were mostly wasted. This is hard to recover from, both mentally and physically. It made me sad to watch him struggle to regain his momentum. If he'd built a foundation of exercise that he could continue at home—or wherever he happened to be—he wouldn't have needed to start again at square one. But the next time he decided to do it the SparkPeople way and was able to build exercise into his lifestyle. Eventually, he went on to help develop the first stage of the SparkDiet.

Joe had gotten caught up in the yo-yo fitness pattern, which is just like yo-yo dieting. It's exactly what I did with my exercise program prior to SparkPeople. And it's what millions of people typically do with both exercise and nutrition. At SparkPeople we pull the plug on this cycle and encourage you to weave exercise and healthy eating right into your healthy lifestyle until you don't even perceive it as a separate component. It simply becomes part of who you are and how you live, as unconscious as brushing your teeth and tying your shoes. Because of all the benefits, we've learned that even very busy people can't afford not to exercise.

Exercise is most powerful when it is integrated into your life in a pleasurable way—as member Shawn tells us:

> It all started with a wedding (my sister's) that got moved up a couple of months. My wife didn't fit into her dress, so she needed to do something fast. At the same time, we discovered that my suit jacket was really tight. She started on SparkPeople, and I just started exercising. After hearing her rave for a couple of weeks, I decided to join up.

I'm the kind of person who really doesn't like the treadmill. Back in June when they were talking about gas prices shooting up again, I decided to give cycling a try. I got my father-in-law's bike for free, used it for a week just for exercise, and then decided to take it a step further. I went out and bought a hybrid cycle and the necessary gear to become a cycle commuter. Now I ride nine and a half miles a day (round trip) to work. In three months' time, I've only had to fill up my car twice, and by the end of today I'll have about 550 miles on my bike. In the last year, I've changed so many things (quiting smoking, eating well and exercising, cycle commuting) that I never thought were possible. SparkPeople has given me the motivation to attack other problem areas in my life to better myself for my sake—and for my family's sake.

One of the huge things that keeps me going is the fact that I have found a way to make exercise fun and save time and money at the same time. I don't dread going to work any more because I know it means I get to ride my bike. I get to exercise, destress, save time, and save money all at the same time.

See and Feel the Results

One reason I love the combination of goal-setting and exercise is that it's so straightforward and tangible, like a recipe: You set a goal, you do the exercise, and after a short time you see and feel the results.

It's such a thrill to feel your body growing physically stronger from your consistent efforts—especially when you understand that this physical strength also translates into mental strength and helps you handle stress. There is even mounting evidence that exercise improves the functioning of our brains.

This is a great way to build momentum, to get excited about going back to the Focus cornerstone and set other goals for your life.

BUILDING BLOCK: NUTRITION

I remember filling up my old car one winter evening with cheap gas and lurching across Cincinnati, my engine knocking away. Sure, my car was old, but filling it with low-quality fuel meant an even more sluggish performance. The same is true with our bodies. Fueling them with empty calories is a sure way to short-circuit our efficiency and power.

People often believe that eating healthy foods means sacrificing everything that tastes good—that they will have to sign on to a monkish life of eating bland gruel. But that couldn't be further from the truth; as you start adopting a healthy lifestyle, your body goes through a metamorphosis. After years of eating greasy fast foods and salty snacks laden with additives and drinking sugary drinks, your poor body has to reacquaint itself with the nuances and subtleties of real food—of how wonderful a fresh berry smoothie tastes, or a muffin baked with whole grains and nuts. Our program includes healthy, delicious recipes for every kind of cuisine and taste—from chicken enchiladas and lasagna to meatloaf, sloppy Joes, and beef stroganoff.

One of the first steps I took when building the nutrition part of the SparkPeople program was to switch from drinking soda to water. In fact, drinking water is one of the best ways to kick-start your healthy nutrition because it's so easy to accomplish and track.

At first, I couldn't stand the taste of water; it seemed so bland compared to soda. Then a funny thing happened. As I stayed with this healthy habit, my tastes began to change and everything turned around. I actually began to enjoy the taste of water and found soda almost sickeningly sweet. Water, however, is a real thirst quencher that the body requires for optimal functioning. Now that it's become my primary drink, I find it so refreshing. This change wasn't a result of "willpower" but a choice my body made. Now it seems ridiculous to drink five or ten teaspoons of sugar (the amount in a single can of soda).

Exercise Your Taste

I know all about poor nutrition—it was my nutrition for years. If we are what we eat, I probably resembled a walking cheeseburger with a side of fries. Even though the food pyramid in our schoolroom called for multiple servings of fruit and leafy greens, in my world it was perfectly possible to go for days without either.

I hated nearly all vegetables. I just didn't like the taste. It didn't matter what I did to broccoli—whether steamed, stir-fried, or boiled—I didn't want any part. But everyone knows veggies are powerhouses of vitamins and nutrients that are necessary for optimum health. But something amazing happened as I became more consistent with my exercise program. I noticed that in addition to craving more water instead of soda, my body now also craved more fruits and vegetables. Most importantly, they actually tasted better! After a workout, I wanted a tangerine or an apple or raw, fresh vegetables, not a greasy serving of French fries. My taste had changed along with my body—and when you consistently incorporate fitness, so will yours.

This is one of the most important components in the SparkPeople System, and the moment when members get it—when they realize that healthy foods really taste better than unhealthy ones and that they prefer them—is one I love to witness. We call this a WooHoo Moment—when a person has taken action and seen results and wants to celebrate.

Think of it as a game: the playing field is your stomach. As you begin to focus on all the healthy, nutritious foods you can eat, they begin to crowd out the unhealthy ones. The bacon cheeseburgers and fries are elbowed out of the way—there's no room for them anymore.

One of the top secrets from our successful members is this: by focusing on drinking more water and eating more fruits, vegetables, and whole grains, they found they didn't feel deprived or develop cravings, like those with a "diet mentality" did. They were less likely to obsess about the foods they shouldn't eat, as member WHGRN60 attests.

> *Last year on Thanksgiving I weighed 286 pounds and was totally out of shape. Ten months on SparkPeople have made a HUGE difference!*
>
> *Today I weigh 188.4 pounds, just 2.4 pounds from my goal! I am the lightest person in my family, instead of the heaviest, as I was most of my life. I am in great physical shape. I work out six days a week and actually enjoy it. Last weekend I did my first-ever 5K walk. It was EASY! And yes, I was at the gym this morning!*
>
> *Tonight I had a great Thanksgiving dinner. I ate exactly what I had planned: turkey, cranberry sauce, stuffing, mashed potatoes, green beans, a piece of bread, and a slice of apple pie. 744 calories. I did not feel one bit deprived. I was quite full actually! I enjoyed the conversation and time with my family, rather than concentrating on food. I am within my calorie range for the day.*

Fit Nutrition into Your Life

I used to find it irresistible to stop at fast-food restaurants on the way home from work. I was tired after a long day and felt entitled to have any meal I wanted. It seemed my car veered automatically toward the golden arches. I deserved it, right? At least that's what I told myself. And since I had no healthy ingredients at home to cook, it was easy to follow my impulse. Of course, I knew the greasy, fat-laden meals weren't good for me, but it was a hard cycle to break.

So I began improving my environment. I shopped for the week and stocked my refrigerator with nutritious ingredients and placed healthy snacks in my car—ones that had a long shelf life, like nuts and raisins. Then when I was driving home and had the urge to stop for fast food, I'd grab a bag of nuts and raisins instead. This was just enough to hold me over until I got home.

This small healthy act, done consistently, made a real difference in my overall nutrition and helped me both physically and mentally. Just as important, I had taken control of this situation and changed a negative into a positive, a downward spiral into an upward one. As time went on, I realized that each time I did this in one small area, it made a real impact in turning my whole life around.

We encourage you to fit healthy diet changes into your lifestyle one at a time, rather than attempting to change everything about your current lifestyle at once. By taking time to take control of your environment, you'll set yourself up for success.

Quick-Fix Society

Our quick-fix society has set us up for failure when it comes to weight loss. We're constantly bombarded with advertising that promises an immediate solution to wrinkles, melancholy, and hair loss, so people naturally wonder, "Why can't I lose weight immediately, too?" Then they sign on to an extreme plan where they lose five or more pounds per week, or they may even turn to diet pills.

The problem is that these solutions don't change your life, even if they do help you lose weight, because they don't change your lifestyle. Typical fad diets are temporary solutions to what, for many of us, is a lifetime problem. Most are based on some kind of calorie deprivation plan. That means that you aren't getting enough calories for your body to function correctly. Sure, you'll lose weight with these diets, but you'll simply regain the weight when you stop because you'll still have the same habits and daily routines that caused the weight gain in the first place. That's why so many dieters gain their weight back within a year. Then they become so discouraged that they gain even more weight and lose even more hope—a classic downward spiral.

Dieting without a lifestyle change is like patching a flat tire. You can put a temporary fix on the damaged area to get the car rolling again. But you'll end up patching it again later down the road—just as you'll probably have to diet again at some point. There are millions of frustrated dieters out there who have made a practice of patching tires again and again, and are still struggling.

Yo-yo dieting might seem harmless, but it's actually dangerous. Studies have shown that yo-yo dieting places a strain on your heart and weakens your immune system. Each time you lose weight and then gain it back, it becomes much tougher for your body to lose weight the next time and much easier to regain it.

Unlike most diets, the SparkDiet is a positive experience. No more yo-yoing here, just steady progress that leads to permanent results.

With all the gimmicky fad diets out there, we've lost sight of the fact that losing weight is usually based on a simple equation: calories in minus calories out.

We'll help you finally master that equation in fun and exciting ways!

And remember, it probably took many years for you to reach your current weight. Doesn't it make sense that it will take time to take it off for good—the healthy way?

In our program, we don't focus on the ten foods you can never eat again or the five foods that you must have every day. Our diet plan encourages variety, portion control, and smart substitutions—small changes that make a big difference.

Our most successful members focus on what they can eat, rather than what they can't—and that includes, in moderation, everything. In fact, we encourage you to eat in order to lose, as member RAYLINSTEPHENS proves:

> The first two months I refused to trust the SparkPeople Nutrition Tracker and logged on my own, but every time I would go below 1,000 calories I would trigger a two to three day binge over 2,300 calories. I lost weight but it wasn't as steady as after I started using the Nutrition Tracker. I had to "let go" and "let Spark" be in charge. I had to trust that I needed to be eating 1,500 calories daily and the weight started dropping. I have continued to average two pounds per week until the last few months where it dropped six pounds and then four pounds per month. But it is still dropping!
>
> My original goal was 165 . . . but I will go as low as my body is comfortable with. We are thinking possibly 125 or even 120?
>
> One day at a time, one pound at a time!

Be Happy, Not Hungry

When people start participating in the SparkPeople online community, they are astounded by the outpouring of positive support from both staff and members. No chiding, no browbeating or negativity—just encouragement, positive thinking, and hope. After the discontents of yo-yo dieting, we often hear that our support system is the most positive they have ever encountered.

Our members have often belonged to other "diet" Websites in the past, and they tell us how negative those online communities can be. Instead of supporting each other, members often tear each other down and even attack newcomers to the community.

It finally dawned on me that most typical diet site communities are full of people following a punitive calorie-deprivation diet, with restrictions, rules, and forbidden zones. No wonder they're grumpy! We know that people who don't eat enough calories become disgruntled for a simple reason—they're hungry!

On the other hand, people who eat enough calories—and understand they are taking the right steps to make healthy, long-term lifestyle changes—are much more likely to be content and happy.

Happy is more sustainable than grumpy. Happy leads to an upward spiral; grumpy leads to a downward spiral.

This is another example of the power of crisscross effects. Following a fad diet or a calorie-deprivation program will make it harder for you to be part of a positive support system. Yet another reason why a healthy lifestyle change is better.

Why not approach weight loss from a sensible, sustainable direction, so you can dump the word "diet" from your vocabulary forever?

The Scale Doesn't Know It All

One of the main frustrations in weight loss is that the scale is often not your friend. You may be working hard, but the scale doesn't seem to notice; the numbers don't budge.

Here's where the tipping-point theory comes into play again. Many people are locked in a desperate, destructive relationship with their scales; if the numbers don't go down, they throw in the towel. This is in spite of the fact that their clothes are fitting better, they're exercising longer, and they feel substantially more fit and alive.

They don't realize that despite what the scale shows, there is real magic occurring inside their bodies that simply takes a while to show up in the numbers.

Member Carol says it best:

> *Kick the scale to the curb! When I first started I was so obsessed with what that scale said! I could see changes, and my clothes were fitting looser, but the scale wasn't reflecting that. When I started measuring and seeing change, it motivated me to keep going.*

We'll show you other ways to measure your progress instead of simply stepping on the scale.

BUILDING BLOCK: STRESS MANAGEMENT

Your body and mind working in tandem are more powerful than you know. That's one reason why stress management is so important at SparkPeople.

When you experience stress, your body releases a hormone called cortisol, which heightens awareness and helps you perform better in "fight or flight" mode. Cortisol was a lifesaver for our ancestors when they were chased through the forest by tigers and bears. But in the midst of modern life, we're not discharging these potent hormones by escaping wild animals. Instead we're becoming overloaded with stress, which causes serious health issues as well as inhibiting weight loss.

The American Institute of Stress has estimated that 75 to 90 percent of all visits to health-care practitioners are prompted by disorders related to stress,[1] and the Mayo Clinic has concluded that psychological stress is the strongest indicator of future cardiac events.[2] Stress is often coupled with poor lifestyle habits such as alcohol intake, smoking, and lack of exercise, which can lead to the hypertension and other illnesses. Just five minutes of stress can leave your immune system vulnerable for nearly six hours.

Stress can also cause you to miss out on opportunities in life. If you have anxiety, you're more likely to hang back, stay on the margins, and avoid trying new things. I know I missed out on many opportunities when I was young because of stress and anxiety. Still, I recognized the silver lining even in this difficult period; without this experience I wouldn't have developed SparkPeople and been able to help so many people seize opportunities in their own lives.

Emotional Eating

At SparkPeople, we often say that what's going on in your head is more important than what goes in your mouth. We've learned from working with millions of people that the number-one reason our members have problems with weight is because of emotional eating.

The SparkPeople program will help you handle emotional eating naturally. As your body grows healthier, you become accustomed to conquering your physical challenges. As you repeatedly set and reach goals, your mind grows stronger. This combination—stronger mind, stronger body—makes you much better prepared to combat the emotional triggers to your overeating. We will also provide you with specific exercises to combat emotional eating. One of these is listing everything in your life that causes you stress, then figuring out how you can either remove or minimize it.

Take Jim, one of our members, who had long been stymied in his weight-loss efforts. A successful electrical contractor, he was a classic Type A personality who spent his life running on adrenaline. He was always on the go, available for faxes, pages, multiple cell-phone calls; he even got up in the middle of the night to check his e-mail. His wife described him as the "white streak," his prematurely gray head canted forward, always rushing somewhere.

Even though he had been jogging on his treadmill every day for half an hour, Jim was still gaining weight and feeling exhausted. It wasn't until he joined our program and began looking at the other facets of his life that he began to see stress's impact.

Jim may have been exercising half an hour each day, but the other 23½ hours were spent in classic workaholic mode. He woke to a blaring radio station delivering a dose of worrisome news, followed by a donut-and-coffee breakfast gulped down in traffic. He spent his working hours dealing with customer demands and tight deadlines. The end of the day was marked by another bout in traffic and then a rushed, solitary meal, long after the rest of his family had eaten. His struggle didn't stop even at night because he suffered from insomnia. He drank beer to relax and often added sleep medication, only to wake up bleary-eyed the next day. Not surprisingly, his fuse was short and his blood pressure was high.

Jim, like so many of us, lived a plugged-in, stressed-out existence. Such chronic coping requires excess physical and emotional energy, which alters the body over time. No wonder weight loss is difficult—it's as if our body is perpetually screaming: "Fire!"

It wasn't until Jim stepped back from his hectic life and addressed his stress that he was able to make meaningful fitness changes that brought the weight loss that had eluded him for so long.

One at a time, he began making small lifestyle alterations. First he began to incorporate shorter and more frequent exercise breaks throughout the day that helped reduce his stress—doing sit-ups and push-ups or taking brisk walks. He sat down and ate a healthy dinner with his family instead of grabbing a pizza on the run. And he learned to unplug at the end of the day, turning off his cell phone and e-mail and playing with his kids so he could relax and get a good night's sleep.

Jim also incorporated one of my favorite stress-reduction techniques—viewing the annoyances of life as challenges instead of stressors. This can completely change how your body reacts to an issue. When he was stuck on a tedious drive, he listened to an audiotape of affirmations; when he found himself waiting for a late client, he jogged around the parking lot instead of fuming alone in his car. He couldn't change the reality of these situations, but he could turn around the way he approached them; rather than experiencing them as stressful obstacles, he altered his response.

In other cases, he was actually able to control the situations that were stress-inducing. Instead of handling the burden of scheduling and paperwork himself, he hired a part-time assistant to do it for him. This freed him from the constant phone calls and online tabulations that interrupted his day. By leaving earlier for work, he began to avoid the traffic jams that jangled his nerves and made him anxious. Both these approaches turned out to be great not just for his mood but for his health. His blood pressure improved, and he began losing weight. He was less anxious, and he found himself slowing down and enjoying the pleasures of his life.

Avoid "Stupid Stress"

I used to be a person who waited until the last moment to leave for an appointment. Since I hate being late, my body was under stress the entire time I was getting ready and traveling to my appointment. This meant that under the best possible conditions I arrived on time but totally frazzled. In the same way, I also waited until the last minute to do homework for classes, putting myself under extreme time pressure to finish—and often ruining a night of sleep. This was stress I was creating for myself, a little furnace I was stoking with my own actions.

Let's face it; we all have enough stress in our lives. The last thing we need is to self-inflict it. I jokingly called this extra pressure "stupid stress" because whenever I was in the thick of one of those situations, I'd say, "This is so stupid!"

Where in your life do you experience stupid stress? How can you prevent it? Here are some systems I have developed:

- Prepare for your morning the night before so you aren't rushed.

- Have simple, healthy snacks both at work and in your car— wherever you might be tempted—to reduce the odds of stopping for unhealthy foods.

- Set up simple fitness equipment so you can always exercise at home.

- Carry extra active clothes in your car in case you get the opportunity to do something fun.

- Look at your goals once a day.

- Set up automatic bill payments to lower the odds of late payments and to keep your credit score high.

- Set up e-mail reminders or a calendar for birthdays, anniversaries, and other important dates, such as car maintenance (tire-pressure check and oil change), home repair (cleaning gutters and furnaces), and routine doctor and dentist appointments.

- Listen to relaxing or motivational music.

- Set up a filing system and file once a week or month, so paperwork doesn't get out of control.

- Start an accomplishments list—ones you worked toward as well as surprise breakthroughs.

My anxiety also created stress because I did silly things under its influence. When I was with a group of people, I'd be so nervous that I often forgot to look around and pick up all of my belongings when I left, thus losing, over time, keys, gloves, glasses, and innumerable pens.

And then there was the time I was driving across town with my friend's stern dad; I was so uptight that I locked my keys in the car when we parked.

This was a small incident, but it made me feel like an idiot. Looking in at the keys behind the plate glass, I realized I had to find some way to prevent this kind of occurrence. From then on, whenever I got up to leave someplace or lock my car, I made myself check out the entire area or look at the key in my hand.

After a while, these small things started to reduce my stress levels by making me feel like I was more in control of my life. I began to have increased confidence. I also started looking at it as a game. Where else in life could I develop smart systems that would make life easier?

BUILDING BLOCK: SLEEP

With the advent of cell phones, Internet, and BlackBerrys, we have become a 24/7 society. This round-the-clock activity often translates into a sacrifice of precious sleep, with the average American getting only six to seven hours a night.

For some reason, getting by with an inadequate amount of sleep has turned into some sort of perverted accomplishment in our culture. At the very least, it's viewed as a necessary evil because of everything going on in our lives. People think they'll be more productive if they sleep less—that they'll be able to fit in more work or play. But borrowing time from sleep is an unwise loan that is difficult to pay back.

Sleep is a time of rest and healing that prepares you for the next day's challenges. A regular amount of sleep brings mental focus and consistency to your program and goals. The more your body gets into the rhythm of regular sleep, the more the rest of your life can find a similar, consistent rhythm.

You may think that it doesn't matter if you skimp on sleep—that you can always make it up later or boost yourself with extra caffeine. But even small amounts of lost sleep add up to a debt that accrues interest, just like on your credit card. Chronic fatigue is simply another anchor, weighing you down, holding you back, and making your body work even harder. This is one of the chief ways people destroy the momentum they've built up toward achieving their goals.

Too little sleep also leaves you vulnerable to stress and raises your risk for depression, anxiety, and cardiovascular problems; it makes it easier to gain weight and harder to lose it. When we're deprived of sleep, our appetites not only increase, but we crave sweets and carbohydrates. In our member survey, we found that self-proclaimed "dieters" slept less on average than healthy lifestylers, who were much more likely to lose weight.

Sleep is also crucial for the proper functioning of our brains. During sleep, our brains are busy consolidating information from our day in an array of amazing functions—reviewing, sorting, organizing, prioritizing, problem-solving, and memorizing. No wonder that a lack of sleep impairs our memory and disrupts our ability to think clearly.

Sleep deprivation also makes you grouchy. When you're in a bad mood, it's hard to be a positive force for yourself, let alone for family, friends, and co-workers.

And finally, lack of sleep can be downright dangerous. The U.S. National Highway Traffic Safety Administration estimates that approximately 100,000 police-reported injuries and deaths per year involve drowsiness or fatigue as a principal causal factor.[3]

Sleep and stress are two building blocks that have strong crisscross effects. Stress can prevent you from falling asleep or lower the quality of the sleep you do get. This, in turn, makes it more difficult to focus on how to reduce stress during the rest of your day.

I'm well aware of all these problems, since I struggled with sleep throughout most of my life. Bed was the perfect place for me to replay the blunders, missteps, and slights that had happened throughout the day. And once I had run through all this, I started worrying about what would happen tomorrow. The possibilities were endless and my worries self-perpetuating. The more I focused on them, the more there seemed to be.

I didn't begin to sleep soundly until the crisscross effects of my self-improvement program began fueling an upward spiral. When I was focused, well exercised, and eating healthy foods, I no longer had the anxiety that had kept me tossing all night. When my mind and body were in synch and at peace, sleep arrived like a welcome visitor to provide me rest and prepare me for a new, hopeful day.

FITNESS FOR LIFE

At some point in our lives, most of us will be confronted with some kind of health issue, ranging from minor inconveniences to debilitating conditions. I personally suffer from terrible allergies, which my younger son has unfortunately inherited. I've watched him sleep many nights when he was so congested that he woke himself up every 5 to 10 minutes.

For the past several years, we—mostly my amazing wife—have had to prepare special meals for him, keep him away from snacks at school, and take him to different specialists in order to find a solution. It has been hard on our family emotionally and physically, but he has been a trouper. Thankfully, in the past few months all the hard work has begun paying off and his allergies seem to be easing. This has improved his sleep and dramatically improved his mood. We feel like we have our son back again. We know we're lucky compared to the challenges other people face.

Meeting the Challenges

From watching my son and hearing from our members, I've seen that no matter the physical or emotional obstacle, there is always the opportunity for renewal and transformation. In the face of every kind of condition, our members have lost weight, gained strength and fitness, and found new joy in their lives. And as a result of our program, the severity of their health challenges has often dramatically diminished. The list of improvements never ceases to amaze me—from lower cholesterol, blood sugars, and blood pressure to the easing of arthritis and the improvement of heart disease.

DIANE_MARY is one of many:

> I went from 145 pounds to 115 pounds in about seven months and kept the 30 pounds off for more than a year now. I eat right and exercise every day. I have myofascial pain syndrome and fibromyalgia so there are many days when working out does not come easy . . . I work out anyway, if I get into my workout and still feel really bad, then I will stop—only then— but at least I know I did my best. Seeing how far I came and how much I am able to work out, despite the fact that my body and mind want to do two different things, makes me feel anything is possible. I am determined to work out and view the myofascial pain syndrome and fibromyalgia as added obstacles I have to overcome. I don't use them as an excuse not to exercise and let them take over my life.

If you are confronted with illness, don't give up. No matter what your condition, a healthy lifestyle will increase your chances of living a more active, vital life. You never know when you'll string together enough small, positive moments to lead to what we call a Breakthrough Point, when incremental change suddenly shows itself in marked improvements—in this case, in your health.

Here's a letter I received from one member:

> I would just like to take this opportunity to thank you for setting up and running this site. It has truly changed my life. About 12 months ago I actually considered suicide. Depression had taken hold. I was agoraphobic and suffered panic attacks. Only my mother convinced me that life was worth living. Refusing medication, I decided to take proactive steps to enable me to start living again, and it was then I stumbled upon SparkPeople.
> To cut a long story short, I now have purpose every day, even if it's a little thing like encouraging someone else on the site. I have made many "friends," who, although I will never see them, make a radical difference to

my life. My confidence has improved to the extent that I recently joined a gym—something I thought was impossible.

I would like to thank you on behalf of myself and my children, who now have a mother who is very much present. You and your team have truly changed our lives.

More Vital Years

There are people who live their lives without ever discovering their real passion or potential because their bodies are sluggish, out of shape, and run down. Fitness helps you live with zest and exuberance. I know *I* want to flourish as long as I can on this planet. Selfishly, I want to be as active as I can to see my two boys grow up. And I want them to have a healthy father and my wife to have a healthy husband.

Wouldn't you love to have more robust, vibrant years to spend with your family and friends, doing the things you love? Being fit won't ensure that you'll reach 100, but it will ensure that the years you do have will be fuller and more alive.

And who doesn't dream of that?

CHAPTER 4

CORNERSTONE:
FIRE

The Pacific Ocean is hardly the most amazing sight I glimpse from my window; even more incredible to me is the natural exuberance of my two young sons. I love to watch them play—how they approach each day with such limitless passion, the way they greet the world with eager faces, how they look up at me and ask, "What's next, Dad?"

At SparkPeople, we call this magic passion *fire.* It's the fuel that turns small sparks into big flames, which creates action and momentum. It's the force that helps you deal with setbacks, stay on course, accomplish your goals, and reach your dreams.

At SparkPeople, we believe that the best time to act like a kid is when you're an adult. We'll help you recapture that inner exhilaration, so that you can look forward to what you're going to achieve, see opportunities around every corner, and live your life with energy and a sense of adventure.

As French military theorist Ferdinand Foch said, "The most powerful weapon on earth is the human soul on fire."

BUILDING BLOCK: PERSONAL LEADERSHIP

Anyone who has ever built a fire knows that it's one thing to start a blaze, but another to keep it going. A fire needs to be carefully built with seasoned wood and well-placed kindling, then lovingly tended until it sparks into crackling flames that burn on their own.

Without such preparations, a fire can be reduced to a smoldering pile of ashes before it has a chance to produce energy and heat.

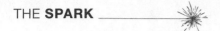

Creating your own internal combustion also requires a firm foundation. You've already begun by focusing on your goals and dedicating yourself to fitness. Now that these cornerstones are working together in an upward spiral, you're ready for personal leadership. Now you can take control of your own life, build your character, and be your own inner motivator, as member Janet describes:

> *I was obese for a really long time. It was a major achievement to get out of the grossly obese BMI range. When I started I was a size 26. The seat belt in my car barely fit. The stairs were a chore. I went out for a walk with friends and couldn't get to the track, let alone take a lap around it. I went to the beach and had a devil of a time getting up a hill from the beach back to the beach house. I dreaded that hill. Hated it. It was the cliffs of Normandy, as far as I was concerned. Then, something happened. I started to work on becoming healthier. I started to track my food, I started to exercise. My mind started to clear. The fog started to lift. I was, suddenly, what's the word? Oh yeah. Happy. I was happy. And I hadn't been that way in forever. I suddenly realized that the seat belt was longer. I went back to that beach, that hill. And I went up and down it a few times. And I was fine. It wasn't a cliff, it wasn't an escarpment. Heck, it was barely a blip. But it was conquered.*

Take Control of Your Life

In my childhood I was so preoccupied with my own anxiety that I spent my days anticipating what might trigger it. Something external, lurking around the corner, was always to blame.

But as I advanced through my self-improvement program, I realized that this was only an illusion. It hit me with particular force one afternoon during the early days of SparkPeople when I found myself standing quite calmly at a podium, preparing to give a speech to over 600 people at a United Way event.

"I'm Chris Downie," I heard myself saying. "Thanks for inviting me."

For someone who'd hidden in books and stared at the ground rather than deal with people, it was hard to believe that I was voluntarily standing in front of this sea of strangers.

In the past, chains couldn't have pulled me onto such a stage. And the 600 people in this auditorium weren't fundamentally different from all the other groups that had terrified me in the past.

I was the one who had changed. I had thought I was protecting myself, but in fact, I'd been holding myself back. Consistently focusing on my goals, pursuing fitness, and

PERSONAL LEADERSHIP ARSENAL

There are many important traits that contribute to being an effective personal leader. Here are some to cultivate:

- *Get organized.* To be in control of your life, you need to be organized with systems in place to help you move efficiently toward your goals and reduce stress.

- *Know how to prioritize.* Learn how to put tasks in the correct order, from most important to least. Otherwise, you may find yourself constantly busy but not moving effectively toward your goals.

- *Stretch yourself but don't break.* When you're building momentum, it's possible to go too far too fast. While it's great to move beyond your comfort zone and try new things, make sure you don't overdo it and lose control.

- *Be a visualizer.* Channel the incredible power of your mind to actually see yourself and your life the way you want it to be. This is a great way to stay on track and reach your dreams.

- *Learn and do whatever you want.* Don't let yourself be placed in a box. Your formal training or job description is only a part of who you are. Don't be afraid to branch out and follow new interests. You never know where a new path might lead you.

- *Don't worry about what other people think.* Don't let other people's views or expectations hold you back from embracing new opportunities. Live your life!

- *Innovate and be creative.* Cultivating the ability to go beyond the traditional ways you've done something can lead to powerful new solutions in many types of situations.

taking action had produced a fire that had propelled me out of the land of anxiety and into a new region, where I was finally free. This was a breakthrough moment, where I punched though a barrier and saw the light on the other side.

Life is the sum of our decisions and actions; results appear where we place our energies. There was no mystery to this, but there was great magic. And look where it had brought me!

The Power to Choose

I had discovered a truth—that the choice to rise to the occasion, to create yet another small victory, or to vegetate and live passively was mine.

Taking control of our lives doesn't mean we will simply sail through our days with our hands on the tiller. As with any great adventure, challenging outside forces will appear along the way. Our challenge is how we handle them.

Consider the example of Christopher Reeve. A near-fatal 1995 horse-riding accident left him paralyzed from the neck down and confined to a wheelchair. Yet weeks after becoming a quadriplegic, he began advocacy work, fighting to increase public awareness about spinal-cord injuries and raising money for pioneering research. Though doctors held no hope that he would ever regain function below the neck, he committed himself to maintaining his body through a five-hour-a-day exercise program, strapped to devices that moved his limbs. He battled infections, broken bones, and blood clots. And for seven years, his body remained motionless.

Yet through steady work and perseverance, by 2004 Reeve had regained sensation in 70 percent of his body, had moved one of his fingers, and had moved his arms and legs in water.

"You can do anything you think you can," Reeve said. "Either you vegetate and look out a window, or activate and try to effect change."[1]

Reeve's inspiring story reminds us that we always have the ability to choose how we respond to life's circumstances—no matter how challenging.

Write to Yourself

Another powerful way to build your leadership skills is by writing in a journal. If you don't already keep a journal, we suggest you buy one now to use at various stages of the Spark program—a simple notebook is fine. As you travel through your adventure, this will help you keep a record of the steps along the way. As Phyllis Theroux writes: "Everybody lives in the middle of a landscape. Writing can provide a map."

By writing down milestones and setbacks, you become more attuned to patterns that might be hampering your progress. Think of the kind of diary you kept as a kid, a place where you're free to dump negative feelings and come up with surprising discoveries. I like to keep a journal and include the highlight of my day each day—or other lessons learned.

In the early days of SparkPeople, we taught a college class at the University of Cincinnati. Each week, we'd assign a journal entry topic based on the SparkPeople System.

I remember reading the journal of a young woman who was simply going through the motions, her writing terse and flat. I could tell she was just trying to finish the assignment as quickly as possible. But as she continued to write and explore her feelings, her tone changed. The pages became filled with new realizations, the writing passionate and alive.

By the end, I could feel the excitement radiating from the page.

"Wow," she wrote. "I'm happy you had us write about this. I've never really thought about this important topic before!"

You'll find it liberating to chronicle how far you've come—as member Diane tells us.

> My life is a 180-degree change from that of three years ago. I've lost 143 pounds and have undertaken new challenges, umpiring high school softball and field hockey. I've taken up golf and biking with my children and have also run two races. I've gone from not getting out of bed until noon to getting up at 6:00 A.M. and heading to the gym every day. I've learned to love exercise and healthy food and believe it all starts with our mental approach. If we believe it we will do it. Tracking food/exercise daily and blogging or journaling about the experience has been so valuable and important. I am constantly amazed at how far I've come and how much better my life has become. I had given up one of my most favorite things in the world—going to the beach—because the last time I had gone I broke my beach chair.

Ultimately, Diane was able to further spread her spark when she appeared on the front cover of *USA Today.*

Build That Character

Character is the foundation of personal leadership, a set of behavior traits—mostly learned—that define what sort of individual you are.

When you set off on a great adventure, you need a compass to guide the way, and that is what character provides.

Developing these traits is key to keeping your fire going and moving you toward your goals. Who knew that good character could help you lose weight? This is an excellent example of how everything in life fits together.

In my case, boldness, optimism, and courage were some of the traits I wanted to develop as I tried to reach my goals.

So how to do it? I began by simply adopting them into my daily lifestyle. When I behaved boldly, suggesting a new idea at work, for example, I found that I liked how it felt so much that I decided to continue using it.

Optimism, one of the most potent of character traits, improves with practice. I focused on the silver lining of challenging situations, the upside of what I'd accomplished rather than how far I had to go. A trait like courage may sound daunting. But you don't have to be a general leading a brigade to exhibit bravery. Holding fast to your goals in the face of adversity involves daily courage—as evidenced by our member Wendy:

> *About a month after I joined SparkPeople, I was diagnosed with breast cancer. Everyone commented on how well I handled the cancer . . . that I always seemed upbeat. I realized recently that I had a secret weapon . . . SparkPeople. Learning healthy methods and watching the scale drop was an excellent distraction from the surgery, the chemo, the hair loss, and the radiation. I kept going to the gym and logging my food the best I could during treatment, and I reached my goal weight in the middle of my chemo.*

You don't need to travel far out into the world to develop these qualities. Practice patience by really listening to a friend or colleague instead of interrupting or tuning him or her out. Cultivate kindness by performing random acts in your neighborhood or community, extending a hand or a listening ear to someone in trouble.

These traits are free to use and easy to practice. Create your own list from the ones below and add traits of your own.

Accountability	Gratitude	Optimism
Boldness	Honesty	Patience
Commitment	Humor	Perseverance
Courage	Initiative	Respect
Enthusiasm	Integrity	Responsibility
Faith	Joyfulness	Tolerance
Flexibility	Kindness	Trustworthiness
Generosity	Loyalty	Wisdom

By developing these qualities, you'll soon find that the powerful leader you're most excited about following is the one embedded in yourself.

BUILDING BLOCK: CONSISTENCY AND MOMENTUM

As a child you probably read Aesop's fable about the tortoise and the hare.

You remember the story—the tortoise won the race by slow, steady progress while the speedy, overconfident hare fell behind because he stopped to boast and take a nap.

This isn't the kind of tale that has much appeal in our culture of instant gratification. We're more attracted to shortcuts—get-rich-quick schemes, instant wrinkle removers, and diets that promise us that we can drop 20 pounds in a week.

But at SparkPeople, we know that slow and steady wins the day. We do sweat the small stuff because we've seen the truth of this ancient fable—that incremental change is far more powerful than any instant-gratification scheme.

SparkStreaks—sustained, consistent acts of self-improvement—are a key element of our fire component. Streaks create momentum that will spread to all areas of your life and keep you energized.

Keeping a streak alive, even for a short time, is an instant power boost. It breeds confidence, builds momentum, and puts you on the winning side again if you're starting to feel yourself slide. It's deceptively simple, but it's proven to work, and that's what counts.

Our member Renay tells us how starting off with her three-times-a-week walking streak helped her forego weight-loss surgery and eventually led to a new life.

> *I started this journey in November of 2005. I am a slow loser, but that is okay because they say the slower it comes off, the easier it is to keep it off. I was at 264 plus. I could not even tie my own shoe. I told my husband I wanted to get surgery, and he said no way. I said, "Fine, I am trying on my own one more time then," and this time it worked . . . I always used to think about how much weight I had to lose, and I would get discouraged so I started only thinking about 10 pounds at a time, and then it started working for me . . . I started out doing 30 minutes of exercise three days a week. Now I do at least 60–90 minutes six days a week, and most days I do even more than that. After a while, things get easier. I am 129 pounds and have lost a total of 135 pounds.*

Another member began her program with a simple streak—cutting out sugary sodas. Most diet plans or self-improvement programs would consider such a small step insignificant. Shouldn't she instead revamp her entire diet and clear her cupboards of all carbs or fats; shouldn't she bounce right off her couch for an hour-long session of kickboxing?

But with SparkPeople, we encourage you to choose an action that you feel confident you can sustain; that's because we know that small successes build a sense of accomplishment and pleasure. Once you've found consistent success in your initial area, you'll discover an inner momentum that is likely to spark success in others.

Sure enough, once our member had refrained from soda for 30 days, she felt such a boost from her own consistency and the fact that she'd lost a few pounds that she was motivated to add another item—giving up potato chips—to her streak and begin to

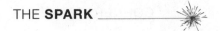

work out at her gym. By 100 days, her continued success made her so enthusiastic that she convinced her boyfriend to start a program of his own. Her personal fire not only lit her own success, but also spread to others.

Consistently building new habits can lead to personal breakthroughs that wouldn't otherwise occur.

We'll give you specific instructions for how to do a streak in Chapter 8.

Get on the Right Spiral

One of the best parts about consistency and momentum is that it helps you get on the right spiral. Imagine this situation: You meet friends at a Mexican restaurant for lunch and end up consuming a plate of cheese nachos as well as a full meal of enchiladas—a calorie count high enough to carry you well through the next day. By the time you get home, you are so upset with yourself that you begin a flurry of negative self-talk that leads you to eat badly for the rest of the day; *I blew it—so it doesn't matter what I do now,* you say to yourself.

Now you feel so rotten that you don't even bother with your planned workout. Then you begin stressing about your diet and worrying about other things in your life. (*I can't follow through on anything—how will I ever lose weight?*) When a family member calls to ask you for advice, you're irritable, and the call ends with both of you frustrated. After you hang up, you head to the kitchen and eat half a bag of potato chips and become even more disgusted with yourself. Finally you go to bed and lie awake ruminating about all the things that went wrong during the day.

This is a common downward spiral. And it began with a few small negative steps that weren't counteracted with something positive, thus souring your whole day. Notice that those original small negative steps had an impact on almost all areas of your life and all four SparkPeople cornerstones. To visualize a downward spiral, think of a kitchen sink where the water is spiraling down the drain—the phrase "it's all going down the drain" is fitting.

Now imagine this carrying over to the rest of the week, as you continue thinking, *Why bother? I can never get this right.* This is a dangerous point because you are now caught in a vicious downward spiral that is hard to stop and can throw you completely off track. The further down you spiral, the more positive steps it takes to bring you back from the edge. After weeks or months of this kind of spiral, some people simply give up.

Depressing, huh? Yet this is exactly how many people live their lives—and it's one of the greatest risks in maintaining a healthy lifestyle. If this is you, I promise you can climb out of this pit. I've been there—as have so many of our most successful members.

Let's go back to the original scenario and turn it around: Instead of getting upset over your Mexican feast, you take two positive steps. First, you realize that you were out with friends and this doesn't happen often, so you say to yourself, *Forget about it, it's only one meal, this is no big deal.* At the next meal you make sure to eat your goal calories and have a few servings of fruits and vegetables. You increase the intensity of your workout and squeeze in an extra 15 minutes, which feels like "extra credit" to you. I call this being an "energy converter," because you've taken something negative and turned it into a positive. Congratulate yourself. You've stopped a potential downward spiral.

Now when your family member calls you're able to give her compassionate support and she expresses thanks for your help. With all of these positive events adding up—especially the great conversation with your family member—you sleep like a baby that night. The next morning you wake up rested and ready to take on the world.

This is what a positive upward spiral looks like, and it can change your life. Let it run as long as you can!

Remember, while it can take many positive actions to dig out of a deep downward spiral, it takes the same amount of work to reverse an upward spiral. The more momentum your upward spiral has, the harder it will be to stop. Negative situations that used to be a real risk will become easier to handle. Once you realize this, you'll have even more confidence.

No matter where you are in life, you can use this energy conversion as a tool. If you're in a low place—if you're depressed, immobilized, or discouraged—you can use it to climb to a brighter spot.

If you already find yourself in a favorable place, this tool can take you to an even greater position. In my case, I was a shy accountant before I developed the SparkPeople System. After an amazing adventure and upward spiral, I'm financially successful, with a wife and two wonderful sons, and I own a company that is helping so many other people reach their goals.

Amazing things can happen to you, too. Are you ready?

Breakthroughs

One of the reasons we focus on taking small steps instead of plowing full steam ahead to reach big goals is this: we know that major life breakthroughs are the result of building consistency and momentum in all four of the cornerstones.

Here are the steps on this continuum:

1. *The Aha Moment.* This is when you realize something for the first time—such as how many calories you consume in a day.

2.   *The WooHoo Moment.* This is when you have taken action and want to celebrate. Maybe it's the first time you've run a mile without stopping and you want to shout "WooHoo!" to the world.

3.   *The Breakthrough Point.* When you string together enough small steps made up of Aha and WooHoo Moments, you start stacking the odds in your favor. Now it's a virtual guarantee that you are closing in on a Breakthrough Point. This could be when you reach your goal of losing 50 pounds and are living a healthy lifestyle. It could be looking great for your wedding. Or, as in my case, it could be reaching a personal tipping point, when all aspects of your program begin working together. A Breakthrough Point is something that can accelerate your life, allowing you to enjoy experiences you may have never thought possible.

On Day 75 of my first fitness streak, I went on a winter vacation with my college fraternity to Jekyll Island, Georgia. The first thing I did after I unpacked was head out to the beach. I stood there a moment, looking out at the ocean, breathing in the salt air, feeling the sun on my face. All at once I began running down the beach, the same sprints I had been doing back home on my asphalt drive. It was such an exhilarating feeling to realize that I was continuing my streak even though I was on vacation. My heart was pumping; the ocean spray was in my face. I felt invigorated and alive. Somewhere along the line my body had begun to crave this kind of physical exertion and pleasure. And I could now count on myself wherever I was.

Sure, I was soon back in my house in cold Cincinnati, doing push-ups and crunches in the early morning darkness. But I had 80 days of success, a storehouse of positive experience behind me that had created an upward spiral. It was a breakthrough when I realized that these new healthy habits were really going to stick this time.

I also noticed a paradox—that the harder and smarter I worked, the more fun I was having. My program had produced so many byproducts, including dramatically increased energy, an understanding of what was motivational and important, and better and deeper relationships with other people.

Because of this, I had more free time to engage in pleasurable activities, there were fewer stressors, and even my work life became infused with passion.

Setbacks—Learn and Get Back on Track

We've been talking about the power of taking small positive steps. But what happens when you have a setback—when you stray from your goals, fall off your exercise plan, or reignite an old love affair with greasy fast food?

Ah, this is one of the most crucial points in staying in an upward spiral instead of falling into a downward one. Many people let setbacks completely derail their efforts. But step back for a minute. If you have one bad day, does it make sense to throw in the towel? To simply let go of all the weeks when you remained on target and focused? Of course not!

At SparkPeople, we use a simple saying to help people handle setbacks: "Two steps forward; one step back." When you have a setback, *choose* to take two steps forward again. Even learning from a setback is considered a step forward! It's okay to make mistakes, especially when you learn from them. The belief that everything should be done perfectly or not at all is the enemy of consistency and momentum.

When you learn to accept that setbacks are a natural part of learning and improving, they are easier to handle. You'll learn much more about this in Week 3 of our 28-day program later in the book.

Overcoming Major Hurdles

These steps will help you deal not only with small setbacks, but also with the major hurdles that eventually come our way, such as health issues, financial troubles, or job loss.

These challenges are obviously much more difficult; often they impact the very fabric of our lives. But as Christopher Reeve proved, you still have the power to choose how to approach them.

Many people who face major hurdles end up becoming even stronger for the struggle. Look at Dara Torres, who came out of retirement in 2008 to win three Olympic medals (added to her previous nine) and become the first swimmer to qualify for five Olympic Games. At age 41, she was 18 years older than the average Olympic swimmer and had also experienced her share of challenges outside the pool. She had known the heartbreak of two divorces (though she's now happily married) and had also struggled with bulimia.

She told a *Time* magazine writer that she wished to convey a single idea: she wanted the middle-aged women who admired her to feel proud of themselves and believe that they could also do whatever they set out to do.[2]

Looking back on my own life, I know that SparkPeople wouldn't exist today if it weren't for my own drive to overcome the hurdles of my early childhood. If you have a major hurdle to overcome, SparkPeople might be able to help you do it much faster than I was able to—that's our goal!

Overcoming hurdles can turn into an advantage for the rest of your life. Many of the people who are most driven to succeed have the experience of overcoming major obstacles. These people learn that once they overcome one major hurdle, they know how to do this again and again.

Take our member Terri:

> *I have Ataxic Cerebral Palsy. When I joined SparkPeople almost two years ago I had no idea of the impact it would have on my life. Not only did I lose almost 40 pounds in 11 months, but with the support of my Spark friends, I am now working on being able to walk with no assistance . . . it's tough, and I'm not quite there yet, but I know I will make it one day. SparkPeople has taught me that not every day will be perfect. The key is to keep moving and not let a few bad days destroy what I've already accomplished.*

People like Terri often make great employees or team members. Why? Because they've "been there, done that." All companies and organizations, at one time or another, will face major challenges, and it's good to have people who have faced adversity before and have come through it successfully. They're ready to face and overcome more challenges. Even if you've never faced adversity in your life, you can replicate the positive effects of it by setting challenging goals and reaching them.

BUILDING BLOCK: MOTIVATION

The legendary explorer Sir Ernest Shackleton's 1914–1916 *Endurance* expedition is one of the world's great survival stories. In 1914, Shackleton and his crew set out from England on a daring mission. His goal was the first crossing of the Antarctic continent, and this was his third attempt. His ship, the *Endurance,* was trapped by ice in early 1915 and then crushed by it ten months later. Shackleton and his men were 1,200 miles away from the nearest outpost of humanity, castaways in one of the most hostile environments on earth. The fact that the crew managed to survive, once Shackleton and five others made a perilous 800-mile journey to get help, is the stuff of legend. His saga of survival for over a year on the ice-bound Antarctic seas is the essence of motivation and passion.

Motivation may be the most powerful tool we possess for reaching goals. It was Shackleton's passion to keep himself and his crew alive that motivated him to cross glaciers on foot and brave the stormy polar seas in an open boat. You may not be involved in an extreme life-and-death adventure, but you have your own journey, which also requires passion and motivation.

Since motivation arises from passion, take a moment and revisit the goals you set in the Focus chapter. If one of your goals is to lose 20 pounds and become healthier, remind yourself why this is so important. Do you want to be a better parent? Do you want to improve a current health issue? Do you want to perform better at work? Knowing why you want to reach your goals will rekindle your passion.

Accentuate the Positive

There is no ally in the world as powerful as yourself.

At SparkPeople we encourage you to view the transformation of your life as an adventure by building a positive, optimistic attitude.

Optimism has a positive impact on both mental and physical health; optimists are sick less often, live longer, and are more successful than pessimists. A positive outlook on life strengthens the immune system, the cardiovascular system (optimists have fewer heart attacks), and the body's ability to handle stress.

Optimists realize that they are responsible for their own destiny. They don't blame themselves or feel victimized when bad things happen; instead they take action. We encourage you to see challenges, not obstacles—possibilities instead of problems. If you lost five pounds in two months and your goal was higher, pick up a bag of sugar and savor what five pounds really feels like—this is weight you're no longer carrying because of your own actions!

According to Martin Seligman, the father of positive psychology, we can control how we think just as we control our muscles. Look to replace automatic negative self-talk, such as *I messed up—I'm a loser,* with a positive alternative: *I had a difficult time today, but I gained new insights from my experience, and I'll be better tomorrow.*

Here's member CASSIOEPIA:

> Change the way you "say" your thoughts inside your head. Self-love is a powerful thing and can really change a person's outlook. When I first started my journey, words like "loser," "lazy," "not good enough" were constantly playing in my head. After some weeks here, they started to play less and less, and now they are mostly gone.

Even a pessimist can become an optimist with enough practice. All you have to do is train your mind to turn in an upbeat direction.

Try some of the following affirmations when you're feeling discouraged:

I'm a survivor.
I am worth the effort it takes to exercise.
I am healthy and strong.

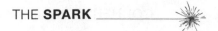

I'm on the path to fitness.
I'm enjoying how I'm feeling now.
I love the feeling of making progress.
I enjoy being healthy.
I'm making things easy for myself.
My body is becoming stronger, slimmer, and healthier every day.
I feel light and joyful.

Our members regularly use such positive self-talk to keep their fire burning. Member Kathy says it well:

> *It's important not to get negative if you make bad choices. Be gentle with yourself. If you know you had a bad day, you are at least paying attention. Figure out why it happened, learn from your mistakes, and do better next time. As time goes by, success breeds success. It's amazing how losing just ten pounds can improve self-confidence and make you feel great! Thinner face, looser clothes, more energy! And oh, the compliments! These have kept me on track through the tough times and plateaus.*

Optimism may take practice, but it's worth it. So why not practice seeing your glass—and plate—not as half empty, but as half full?

Make It an Adventure

Many people approach changing their health habits from a position of pain. They nag and berate themselves and expect nothing less than perfection. If they aren't comparing themselves with others, they're judging themselves harshly. Guilt, doubt, shame, and self-flogging are common tools of this trade. Instead of celebrating the 24 pounds they've lost, they only see the 6 they still have to lose. Does this sound familiar? If you're accustomed to beating yourself up, it may seem like the best way to get motivated. But consider this: If you attempted to motivate employees this way, how long do you think they'd stick around? How successful would they be?

The world is hard enough, so let's try it differently this time. Approach your goals from a position of possibilities instead. Find ways to use regular rewards to pat yourself on the back. Treat yourself with compassion. When you have an off day, reset your counter and try again. Instead of focusing on what you do wrong, pay attention to what you do right.

Our motto at SparkPeople is "Make Your Life an Adventure." That's why our program turns the pursuit of a healthy lifestyle into an exciting undertaking, with plenty of pleasure and rewards. Remember: it's not just about the destination, but also your journey along the way.

As in the case of our member JSCHARF, a beloved child can play the role of goal buddy, providing courage and hope as your adventure unfolds:

> *Children are amazing. When I started out with SparkPeople back in July of '08, I enlisted the help of my family. My seven-year-old daughter has been there for me when I have least expected it, motivating me and making a difference in my life.*
>
> *Yesterday we went out on our first family "jog." I ended up going a little slower because my daughter was with me. During the jog around the subdivision, we talked about the tortoise and the hare fable where "slow and steady wins the race." Amazingly, we did one lap around the subdivision.*
>
> *What was even more surprising was that she wanted to do another lap! We kept jogging and motivating each other by saying "slow and steady . . ." as well as "we can do it!" (my daughter's favorite saying). When we finished, 25 minutes had gone by and our arms were outstretched in victory!*
>
> *This was a huge moment for me, because when my daughter was born, she had a double hip dysplasia and had to wear a harness for the first nine months of her life. She had no hip sockets for her leg bones to go into. After months of therapy, she could walk as a toddler. Now at seven, she is an athlete who loves soccer and is very active. My daughter is also mentally tough and always tries her best. If a girl who had hip dysplasia can keep up with her dad and finish the "race," then losing weight and keeping fit for her dad should be really easy in comparison.*
>
> *I can truly say that one of the best moments of my life was finishing that run and hoisting my daughter into the air . . . if she can do it, anybody can!*

Hold On to Your Inner Child

Children have so much to teach us. Their abundant passion and joy remind us how to savor life. By combining the wisdom of an adult with the joy of a kid, you now are in the position to approach your goals with a new sense of adventure and fire.

The next time you watch children play, as I watch mine—appreciate their natural inner passion. Then take another step—go outside and join them. Seize the day! This is your chance and your life!

CHAPTER 5

CORNERSTONE: POSITIVE FORCE

You may not be accustomed to thinking of yourself as wealthy. But by the time you've reached the fourth cornerstone of the Fuel for Improvement journey, you are the beneficiary of an inner richness that no stock-market plunge can take away.

Using the first three cornerstones, focus, fitness, and fire, you have amassed a new abundance. Now you'll discover a surprising new impulse—you'll want to start giving some of it away.

There is a feeling of satisfaction and fulfillment unlike any other. It doesn't come from winning the sweepstakes or buying a yacht and the side effects don't include buyer's remorse or an empty wallet. Have you ever felt it?

It comes from contributing your time and energy to something greater than yourself, from using the power of your own personal transformation to impact the lives of others.

In our program, this component is called *positive force.* We know that the action of any one of us has the potential to impact everyone. Just as the flapping of a butterfly's wings can influence the formation of a far-off storm, our most seemingly insignificant acts can have powerful consequences. As you achieve goals and live with passion, you'll end up impacting more people than you know.

AN ENERGY MULTIPLIER

People tend to think of energy as a finite resource that can be depleted, like money. But in reality, giving is an energy multiplier. The more you spend, the more you have. And when you invest outside yourself, the dividends not only enhance your internal portfolio but spread to improve the lives of others.

Acting as a positive force builds a confident new self-image fueled by the transformational power of personal change. You not only remain committed to your own goals, but you refocus your sights: you have more, you give more, and you reach even higher.

I became aware of the reciprocal nature of positive force through my encounter with Pat, my co-worker at P&G. As I worked to keep my fitness streak alive, I was unwittingly inspiring Pat, sitting across the hall from me, to embark on a self-improvement program of her own.

Her words—"Chris, you changed my life"—altered my perspective and made me realize that we never know the impact our smallest actions have on others. This was doubly true when I learned that Pat was spurring other people on to do the same.

That encounter started a chain reaction that still reverberates today. Whenever I read grateful letters from such far-flung places as Japan or Alaska, from people who have dropped a hundred pounds or jogged across a finish line for the first time, I am humbled and awed by how that single encounter in my Cincinnati office sparked a grassroots movement of millions of people who have transformed their lives. Acting as a positive force is how you spread your fire and take your program to another level.

At SparkPeople, we look for opportunities to cultivate positive force in several areas: coaching, public leadership, and community service.

BUILDING BLOCK: COACHING

Coaching is a special type of public leadership, with several potent variations. You can be someone's coach, you can be coached by another person, and you can even coach yourself. This is why we make it a building block in the Positive Force cornerstone.

Role Models—Your Coaches

How do we learn to lead our lives? First from observing our parents, then by widening the net and following the lead of those whose lives and accomplishments we admire. We all need role models for inspiration and guidance. As examples of passion and purpose, they're living proof that excellence can be pursued and greatness can be accomplished. Role models are all the coaches you've had in your life. Some of them may be extremely close to you; others you may have talked to only briefly or never even met.

One of the most influential in my life was John Pepper, the former CEO of Procter & Gamble, a charismatic leader who didn't fit the stereotype of a CEO.

He was named chairman during my tenure; I remember the annual meeting where his position was announced, held in a huge sports arena in Cincinnati. I was one of the

10,000 people who attended the event and gave him a standing ovation, a response usually reserved for rock stars and sports heroes. Later, when I attended an event for new hires, he approached our table and spoke to each of us with ease and charm.

"My wife's out of town so I'm making my own dinners, too," he said with a smile before he walked off.

Here was a powerfully important man with such a natural, humble manner that his employees wanted to do their best. I wanted to be like him, to find a way to empower and motivate people, not intimidate them.

In his book, *What Really Matters*, Pepper quoted a passage from the Talmud that stuck in my mind: "You are not required to complete the work, but neither are you free to desist from it."[1] Pepper's example, the way he stressed community service, diversity, and innovation, lodged in my consciousness and stayed there, long after I left P&G and he went on to become the chairman of the board of Disney. When I imagined my own future, and who I would be in it, I found myself consciously trying to adopt his traits. This is what role models do for us—they provide a blueprint, a path that we can follow, as we forge our own way. They serve as reminders that we too can achieve great things.

Bell's theorem is a theory in science that claims that two particles, once connected, are never separated, but forever stuck together by something called space entanglement. I sometimes think of this with John Pepper—that a bit of him is somewhere embedded in me and what I've tried to do.

One of the smartest strategies you can use to become a positive force is to search for positive role models and coaches. In this way, you'll be "standing on the shoulders of giants," learning from those who've come before you, taking their teachings and example to another level.

President Obama's role models include his late grandmother Madelyn Dunham, who was credited for her accomplishment, humility, and strength. After her death, he remembered her as "one of those quiet heroes we have across America, who aren't famous . . . but each and every day they work hard. They look after their families. They look after their children and their grandchildren."

That definition could fit so many around us.

Another important role model and coach for me was Rob, my original partner at Up4Sale. I remember observing how proficient he was at attacking new skills. Even though he was an accounting and finance major in college, he sat up late at night learning computer programming, a valuable skill that enabled us to build our own Website. His initiative inspired me to follow his example. Although I was acting in our new company as the accountant, my mind was full of ideas for how to advertise and broaden our brand. Rob's example made me realize that I didn't have to narrow my focus to only one skill set. If he could branch out, why couldn't I? So in effect I also became our marketing department.

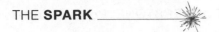

I was able to draw on the real-world marketing expertise I'd learned from starting a small T-shirt company in college. In the end, I figured out several innovative online marketing strategies that led us to gain nearly $10 million in marketing value for almost zero actual cash. Rob's leadership initiative sparked mine.

Once you've identified your role models take a moment and note the positive qualities that you find so inspiring. Then look inside and identify what qualities you already possess. For example, I already shared John Pepper's humility, but it was his charisma and leadership skills that I particularly wanted to emulate.

Then locate the traits you don't yet possess. If your role model is an inspiring speaker, consider taking a public-speaking course or finding opportunities to practice this skill. Emulate your role model; adopt his skills and habits, but always do it in an authentic way that is true to yourself.

This will boost your self-confidence, spur you on to new goals, and make you want to reach even higher.

Pass It On—Be a Coach

In all of time, there will never be anyone just like you. You're unique not just in your DNA but also in your talent and wisdom. So why not take your special expertise, your unique fingerprint, and pass it on? If you don't believe you possess a special talent, look again. Embedded in your life right now are valuable experiences and skills. If you know how to plant a garden, file a tax form, write a resume, or drive a car, you have an asset to share.

As a reader, you can help a student complete a GED or apply for citizenship. If you know how to use a computer, you can pass on your knowledge to a young person or a senior.

And don't forget your spark. Working closely with another person to develop his or her spark can inspire both of you to reach new heights. There are millions of people who don't know how to live a healthy lifestyle. They haven't mastered the skills you've learned from reading this book—such as the smart way to set and reach goals. In fact, going through the SparkPeople program prepares you to become a great coach. You might be able to help close friends and family members—or even complete strangers. We had a member who told us that she was standing in Walmart looking at fitness equipment when a person she'd never seen before came up and began to tell her about SparkPeople. Our program encourages members to use their life experiences to coach each other, as member Kimmie writes:

I am training to become a Spinning instructor, and soon I plan to be a personal trainer. I feel since I have been down this road I can relate so well to other people. I truly know what it is like to be so overweight, and I would love to help people accomplish their dreams and goals! I have come so far on this weight-loss journey, and from time to time I remind myself that I don't ever have to go back. I get to be the new Kimmie for the rest of my life, the healthy and fit girl!

BUILDING BLOCK: PUBLIC LEADERSHIP

By now, you've learned how to focus, take responsibility, and build character in constructing your personal leadership foundation in the Fire cornerstone. In fact, skills learned in all three of the other cornerstones will also prepare you to become a strong public leader.

Public leadership isn't some secret skill reserved for corporate boardrooms or political office. A leader is anyone who lives according to his core principles and elicits the best from others. As leadership expert Lance Secretan writes: "Leadership is not a formula or a program, it is a human activity that comes from the heart and considers the hearts of others. It is an attitude, not a routine."

What Makes a Leader?

Good leaders inspire by word or deed. They involve others and build teams around common ideas, whether in the office, on the battlefield, or at home. They have the opportunity to bring people together to find solutions, thus transforming potential negative situations into positive, empowering outcomes. Take the recent case of Paul Levy, CEO of Boston's Beth Israel Deaconess Medical Center, which was faced with laying off employees because projected revenues were far below projected costs. Levy confronted the problem head-on at an employee meeting. Stating that he didn't want to have to lay off anyone, he asked the hospital employees for ideas and solutions. According to an article in *The Boston Globe,* "The consensus was that the workers don't want anyone to get laid off and are willing to give up pay and benefits to make sure no one does. A nurse said her floor voted unanimously to forgo a 3 percent raise. A guy in finance who got laid off from his last job at a hospital in Rhode Island suggested working one less day a week. Another nurse said she was willing to give up some vacation and sick time. A respiratory therapist suggested eliminating bonuses." Levy said he was receiving nearly a hundred messages per hour with ideas.[2]

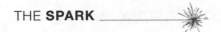

That is what great public leaders can do—transform challenges into successes.

Public leadership has played a major role in my own journey. I had a boss from P&G named Dave Raichle who inspired me without even realizing it. Although he arrived in our department after it was already established, he authentically cared about the success and performance of our team rather than simply striving to gain credit for himself.

I admired his innovative spirit and boldness, the way he came up with a program and direction—seemingly out of thin air—then said, "Let's try it!" I was accustomed to sitting through meetings and long, drawn-out discussions, but Dave came up with an idea—or listened to someone else's—and then presto! we were working as a team to implement it.

This had a huge impact on me. I realized that great public leaders rally their teams, no matter how large or small, to get things accomplished. Now that I'm an entrepreneur with my own blank slate in front of me, I often follow Dave's lead and toss out a new idea and make a commitment to action—as well as listen for good ideas from other team members.

There are many important skills involved in being a great public leader. Here is a list of some of the top ones:

- A solid personal-leadership foundation
- Listening and empathy
- Teamwork—including recruiting great people to the team
- Delegation—including finding the right role for each team member
- Motivating others
- Getting results
- Leading by example
- Giving credit appropriately to team members
- Helping team members improve their skills
- Public speaking

The first skill—having a solid personal leadership foundation—may be the most crucial of all. In order to stay on a positive path, you need to evaluate the leaders you choose to follow. People who have great public leadership skills but "faulty" personal leadership skills are people to avoid.

And Remember . . .

While you're leading an inspiring life, someone is watching. When you build a team, take initiative to solve a problem, or confront an issue, you're spreading a positive force that will be picked up by others who emulate your actions. Our member DOGGY says it well:

> Take the time to encourage other people along the way. Take risks; open yourself to new possibilities and relationships. That's what SparkPeople is all about. You can be an inspiration. Think about that. You are an inspiration. One day someone will tell you that you inspired them, and it will make you feel great.

BUILDING BLOCK: COMMUNITY SERVICE

Herman Melville wrote: "We cannot live for ourselves alone. Our lives are connected by a thousand invisible threads, and along these sympathetic fibers, our actions run as causes and return to us as results."

Community service, the final component of positive force, is based on the old epitaph: "What I gave, I have; what I spent, I had; what I kept, I lost."

Serving others is one of life's greatest enrichers. It provides purpose and meaning, allows you to spread your fire, and gives you a new perspective. Whether it's helping an elderly neighbor, volunteering at a children's hospital, helping students learn to read, or cleaning up trash in your neighborhood, the most effective community service is rooted in action. With more energy and motivation from the other three cornerstones, you might find that you now have more time to be part of your community in ways that will enrich your life.

Doing Good Is Good for You

Volunteering and community service can reduce isolation and boredom, boost mood, and foster a feeling of belonging. With more than 10 percent of men and women across the nation taking antidepressants, volunteering and community service may be the cure for what ails so many of us. And Martin Seligman has done research that shows that meaningful engagement is what leads to long-term happiness—the fulfillment you gain when you're engaged in an effort that is greater than yourself.[3]

Aside from this incredible positivity that can fuel everything you do, community service also gives you the opportunity to meet new people, enhances your social support network, and provides you with new skills and opportunities that you can use for your career. And, as our Secrets of Success member survey indicates, helping other people can help you be more successful across the board.

In our survey, we asked people to rate how important it is to them to help other people; in another question, we identified people who regularly reach out to other members to encourage them on their journeys toward their own goals. The people who spent more time helping others actually had a slight edge on the rest of the population when it came to reaching their own goals, whether it was reaching their weight-loss goals, feeling more confident, or reporting higher levels of happiness—anywhere from a 5 percent to a 10 percent advantage!

Newton's third law of motion states that for every action there is an equal and opposite reaction. Service to others is more than a two-way street, it is a busy intersection with crisscross effects that help not just the receiver but also the giver.

In a study at Johns Hopkins University of older adults who participated in a volunteer program with students at troubled urban schools researchers found that while the volunteers were improving the educational outcomes for teens, they were also boosting their own mental and physical health, lowering their blood pressure, and strengthening their immune systems.[4]

A volunteer experience changed my life; it was a trip I took with my future wife's church to a remote Mexican village that rarely saw outside visitors. Despite living conditions that seemed rustic to us—we slept in hammocks in a thatched-roof hut and shared a single communal bathroom (where we had to make sure there weren't scorpions before we sat down)—these villagers exhibited a sense of community cohesiveness and cooperation that made a deep impression. I remember watching older children attend to a group of toddlers with great tenderness and care. I got the sense that everyone looked out for one another, that they were all united for the common good of their village. So while we went there to help them put a new roof on their church, *they* inspired *me* by their example. I saw that what we can accomplish together is far greater than what any of us can do alone.

A Sparked Community

The warm camaraderie and interconnection I'd witnessed inspired me to make community support a central component of our program. At SparkPeople we know that people are nurtured and bolstered by a close, caring environment. Our experience has shown us the power of connection, of members listening to each other and saying, "Yes, I hear you. I know how you're feeling. You're not alone."

Unlike other programs that focus solely on diet, we offer wide-ranging opportunities for spreading positive force and building supportive community, online and offline. Our members aren't banding together simply over weight but also over health issues, fitness, hobbies, careers, parenting, even pets.

One of these community groups, the 100 Plus Club, has helped members lose more weight than they ever dreamed possible. Here's Dorothy on her experience:

I started SparkPeople due to a very high cholesterol level and my doctor wanting to put me on medication. I was unwilling to do this, so I knew I had to find something. I found SparkPeople. Joining the 100 Plus Club was the best thing that happened to me. I started posting and in a very short time members were encouraging me, cheering me on. I never had felt such support. They understood the feelings and problems that come with needing to lose 100 pounds. My first year I had lost 65 pounds and was now walking, taking swimming lessons, and kayaking—all at 40 plus years old.

LEAVE YOUR MARK

Imagine being part of a movement of millions, all striving to act with positive force. Every small step and major breakthrough you achieve contributes to a dynamic and uplifting spirit—one that has the power to change the world.

While you may never realize the impact of the encouragement you've offered or the hand you've outstretched in support, there are times when the results are dramatically apparent, as in the case of our member Linda.

Linda spread her positive force by convincing her husband, Dave, to join Spark-People with her and embark on a new lifestyle of exercise, healthy eating, and smoking cessation. Months later, when Dave suffered a serious heart attack, the doctors credited his improved fitness for his survival.

Here is Linda:

Dave is still with me, but we came very close. His heart stopped ten minutes after I got him to the emergency room and then again on the operating table. But they've placed a stent in the right coronary artery that opened things up again. He has a lot of heart damage due to both the stoppages and the electric shocks to restart the heart, but we'll deal with that.

The medical team, including his cardiologists, nutritionists, and cardiac rehab group, were very impressed with the SparkPeople site and the nutrition guidelines. We were amused to learn that his "new, heart-healthy diet" prescribed by his medical team was actually the diet he has been following on SparkPeople for the past several months! I linked all of them to the site and they told us to keep on doing what SparkPeople was recommending in

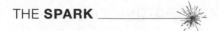

terms of his nutrition guidelines, water intake, and exercise, in addition to the new cardiac rehab program.

Today he wore his SparkPeople T-shirt, so he had lots of opportunities to "Spread the Spark," although I was doing all the talking!

Thank you! If we had not started following the SparkPeople programs, reading articles, and generally changing our lifestyle over the past several months, I would very probably have lost my best friend in the world.

And from her husband, Dave:

There can never be words to express the gratitude I have felt over the last week to Spark members and others in the community who supported me and more importantly Linda. I have had friends say things like, "I don't get it, you are in great shape, you eat right . . . But I can hear the words of my surgeon who helped save me from death several times—if my heart had not been in pretty good shape, along with the diet and exercise regimen my wife had inflicted on me, I would not be here.

Linda and Dave's story is pretty dramatic. But remember that being a positive force doesn't have to entail drastic sacrifice, a long-term commitment, or becoming involved in a complicated process. Every day, with each interaction you make, you have a chance to make a difference in the world.

Simply look around—there are opportunities everywhere.

Welcome a newcomer to your block or take library books to a homebound person. Hug someone who's having a hard day. Spread sunshine by offering the freest and easiest of human expressions—a smile.

As you perform these simple acts, you'll realize the most profound of truths—that what we do matters.

PART II

THE SPARKDIET

So many people come to SparkPeople longing for a different way of life. Some arrive carrying lots of extra weight, as well as the additional burden of years of failure. They come to us with a mixture of promise and trepidation—half daring to hope, half frightened to try. *Can this program really work and be different?* they wonder. Yet once they launch into our program and make small, steady steps on their own behalf, hope and excitement begin to build again. Their misgivings, fear of failure, and lack of confidence start to recede. They begin to feel in control again as they take back their own lives. This is an exhilarating moment. And it's a thrill for me to witness what is often the beginning of an exciting and powerful transformation.

In these early weeks, we often hear members report that they have started to feel successful, even before the scale starts to move. They tell us "it's different this time" and "this time I know I can do it." Like our member 2CATCRIB, who came to SparkPeople believing she would be overweight forever, but went on to meet her goals. "SparkPeople gave me my confidence back, even before I met my goals. SparkPeople helped me understand that taking action *is* success."

That's exciting to hear because I know what lies ahead for these members—if they continue to persevere, this feeling will grow with each small step they take and each milestone they reach.

Take THINMOM5, who has reached her final weight goal and has stayed at this weight for almost a year:

> As much as I've enjoyed the physical makeover, I'm most pleased with the makeover I've felt on the inside. I've always considered myself a confident person, but SparkPeople took that to a whole new level. I know that if there's something I want to achieve, I can. If there's a mountain I want to climb, I can do it.

Now it's time for you to get started—to convert the inspiration from the first half of the book into action that will change your life. It's time to let *your* spark grow into a mighty flame!

THE BIG PICTURE

I developed the SparkPeople System as a philosophy to help ordinary people achieve their goals and even radically transform their lives. This philosophy shows you how everything fits together and is connected by crisscross effects that reach through all areas of your life, making each stronger and more powerful.

But I also wanted to build a step-by-step practical program so people could put this way of thinking into action. The SparkDiet is a program that helps people make the elusive jump from dieting to a fresh new healthy lifestyle—one step at a time.

With the SparkDiet, this shift to a new healthy lifestyle happens in four stages.

Stage 1 (Fast Break) is a warm-up that helps you shift your mindset from the old diet mentality to a new way of thinking. This is a critical stage that lets you experience success again, an important motivator to propel you on your journey. In Stage 1 we help you take small steps to build early momentum. We call these steps "Fast Break goals," and they are simple and easy yet incredibly powerful. This first stage puts you on track to change your life!

In Stage 2 (Healthy Diet Habits), SparkPeople acts as your coach to help you learn core healthy habits and make one lifestyle change at a time. These habits form the foundation of good health and lasting weight loss.

In Stage 3 (Lifestyle Change), you learn how to be your own coach, a crucial skill to sustain a healthy weight and make a lifestyle change last forever. You discover what truly motivates you, learn how to handle setbacks, and surround yourself with ways to stay motivated no matter what happens.

Stage 4 (Spread the Spark) is not the end, but the beginning of living a sparked life. In this stage, you (1) spread the spark to other people—a great way to keep yourself on track and be a positive force to others—and (2) spread your spark in your own life by setting and reaching goals in other areas. This stage is where you are reminded that getting fit is not an end in itself, but rather a springboard to help you live to your fullest potential.

THE 28-DAY PROGRAM

In this book, we've taken our 12-week online program and for the first time distilled the best core principles into a 28-day program meant to spark your life and get you moving toward your goals. This is a flexible, easy-to-follow plan that is accessible for people at any level—from those new to SparkPeople to experienced members who want new sources of motivation. You'll be able to work at your own pace. You can advance through the stages quickly, take your time, and go back to review whenever you feel the need. Each week, you'll add action steps from one of the four stages so that you'll begin to experience the key habits and behaviors that will lay the foundation for success and sustain you once you've reached your goals.

The combination of action steps in a manageable time frame will help you create new habits that stick. The small steps you take in Stage 1, the first seven days, help you break the inertia, experience success, and retake control of your life. The following 21 days of consistent action are designed to help you form healthy habits that will last for life. If you can rise to the challenge of 21 days of these consistent actions, you will feel more energy, lose weight, and create a momentum that will let you spring forward toward your goals and a new sparked life.

By the end of your time on this program, you'll never need to "go on a diet" again. By then you'll realize that traditional diets are an outmoded concept, destined to fail in most cases. Instead, you will be a SparkPerson, ready to reach amazing goals you never thought possible!

SPARKPEOPLE DVD

At SparkPeople, we believe exercise and weight loss should be enjoyable. That is why we are always coming up with new and innovative approaches that make living a healthy lifestyle fun and easy. To give people more options for quick workouts that fit the SparkPeople 28-day program presented in this book, we created a DVD called *The Spark: Fit, Firm & Fired Up in 10 Minutes a Day*. You don't need this DVD to do the program in the book, but it's a great additional resource if you like to work out at home. It includes seven 10-minute strength workouts, plus a bonus cardio workout, all of which can be mixed and matched to make longer workouts.

SPARKPEOPLE EXPERTS

SparkPeople has put together an amazing team of experts who are passionate about helping people reach their goals. This team includes registered dieticians, personal train-ers, and behavioral psychology experts. Coach Nicole, Coach Dean, and Coach Becky have all helped significantly with the expert information for this book and you can see them regularly on the Website along with me.

We also feature advice and comments throughout this book from our Community Team members. The Community Team is a group of more than 3,000 people from around the world. These are actual SparkPeople members who came to the site to lose weight or get fit and have now become team leaders, helping other members with their motivation and knowledge. Leading teams and working so closely every day with mem-bers gives the Community Team firsthand perspective on what works, as well as fun ideas to make things stick.

In this second part of the book, our entire team of experts and community leaders will now be working with you, as well as our millions of members, who'll continue to share their personal experiences. By successfully traveling the road themselves, many of our members have become "everyday experts" who can give other travelers tips about what lies ahead and how best to navigate the path. I am continually amazed and thankful for their dedication to reaching goals and helping others.

MAKE IT A GAME

Since the core program is in part based on results from our Secrets of Success survey, we know it truly works and has already transformed the lives of thousands of people and helped them reach their goals. Now it's your turn!

One secret many SparkPeople members use to stay motivated is making healthy activities into a game. Almost half of our successful members use some form of competi-tive activities as motivational tools, and many of them monitor their activity levels by keeping track of SparkPoints on SparkPeople.com.

We designed SparkPoints to encourage members to perform activities and tasks that are proven to help them reach their goals. SparkPoints can be earned for almost every healthy activity—whether walking, doing strength training, tracking food, or even participating in the online community to support others. Each healthy action you take helps you increase your points. For anyone into video games, you know how motivating it is to watch your score go up! And if you join a SparkTeam, you can start to see how your score measures up against other teammates. All part of healthy and friendly competition. Many members say they didn't realize they were competitive until they started earning SparkPoints.

With SparkPoints, you have a choice. You can go online and use the special part of the SparkPeople.com Website that follows along with the book. Or you can use the version of SparkPoints that is fully outlined in Appendix E. SparkPoints are a great way to motivate yourself to actually do the activities that are key to changing your life. I currently have 30,000 SparkPoints. How many can you earn? Give it a try; you might be surprised at how well this works!

Now is your time!

CHAPTER 6

STAGE 1:
FAST BREAK

Our bodies are complex, intricate miracles, each as singular as a snowflake, composed of histories, life experiences, and genetics that are unique. That's why approaching weight loss from a narrow, one-size-fits-all perspective is so frustrating—and often futile.

But at SparkPeople, we know that you encompass more than the flickering numbers on a scale. We focus on the full breadth and scope of your life in order to help you reach your potential.

At 39, our member Sue had tried most of the popular diet programs—zones and points, fat blockers and calorie deprivers—and had never lost more than a few pounds. At 218 pounds, she now had arthritic knees and rapidly vanishing self-esteem. She still had a vision of herself being a fit and active person again, who could ride a bike, feel confident, and commit herself fully to her career as a social worker. But that vision was growing dimmer.

Like so many people who join SparkPeople, her flame of hope was nearly extinguished. When she found our program, we told her something she had never heard before: "You can do this! Our plan is different. We'll help guide you, one small step at a time."

We came up with the Fast Break as a method to get people like Sue immediately engaged and light their sparks again—to give them a taste of success and a flicker of hope that this time they can succeed.

Just as an athlete requires preparation before taking the playing field for an important game, we helped Sue take time to prepare to make a healthy lifestyle change. We assisted her in focusing on her true reasons for wanting to lose weight. We helped her gather the right equipment and prepare her environment. We guided her on how to be mindful of eating habits, triggers, and the reasons behind them. We gave her inspirational tips to keep her true goals in sight.

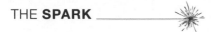

This approach got her off the couch, sparked her motivation, and connected her with others who cheered her on. A year after starting our program, she's now an active 162-pound woman on a five-speed, working with autistic children in a job she loves. And she began one small step at a time.

WEEK 1 ACTION STEPS

For you, as for Sue, this is a chance to transform your life. In the Fast Break, we'll ask you to take six action steps so you are completely prepared for the coming adventure. Those action steps are to:

1. Set your Fast Break goals
2. Plan your SparkTime
3. Reaffirm your focus
4. Set up shop
5. Choose your rewards
6. Learn about what you currently eat

At the end of this week, you'll even earn a small reward for completing these activities!

SET YOUR FAST BREAK GOALS

For the Fast Break stage, we ask members to set and track three small goals—ones that might seem inconsequential. For example:

"Can you eat one fruit and one vegetable on at least five of the next seven days?"

"Can you do ten minutes of exercise on at least five of the next seven days—even if it's as simple as walking around the block?"

"Can you write one page in a journal on at least five of the next seven days?"

The goals are designed to be so simple that the only possible answer is, "Of course I can!"

Sue accomplished these goals by adding an apple and a salad to her menu each day; she got up in the morning and walked two blocks to the post office and back; and she bought a spiral-bound notebook and wrote a page about her feelings each evening before she went to bed. That's it!

These activities took less than an hour of her day. Yet meeting these small goals was the first time in years she had consistently followed through on a commitment to herself. This single week created tremendous excitement and a sense of accomplishment in her. By building confidence one step at a time, these simple acts of goal achievement whetted her appetite for more.

The power of consistently setting and reaching small goals is one of the most magical parts of SparkPeople and makes a Breakthrough Point—when something incredible happens—almost inevitable. And that breakthrough could happen in any of the building blocks of the four cornerstones.

But the key is getting started. Members who take this "small continuous steps" strategy seriously often end up being the most successful. We hear many stories of people who started by walking a quarter mile on a gravel road and ended up running a marathon or losing over 100 pounds.

The Fast Break stage is an important springboard that provides power to the weeks ahead. Of all the steps and strategies, we think this part is often the most crucial. Many people, like Sue, become excited when starting a new program, but they set goals the wrong way, paving a path to failure instead of success. That's why we want to spend time helping you get this first step right.

Start Small to Achieve Big Results

Don't worry if you think these steps are too small to be effective. According to our Secrets of Success survey and what we've seen in thousands of members' lives, we know that this somewhat counterintuitive approach works in losing weight.

Almost 80 percent of successful members start small, with little steps, and once they build a firm foundation, they move on from there. Those in our survey who called themselves "dieters" were more likely to start with big goals, and go all out trying to lose weight fast—only to fail, often repeatedly.

Small steps not only lay a firm foundation of success and confidence when you're starting out but also make it easier to recover when you've had a setback. You can easily return to small steps to get back on track, another key to successfully losing weight and living a long-term healthy lifestyle.

Providing yourself with opportunities for small successes gives you hope and confidence, which creates the momentum and drive that fuel your pursuit of goals. Sue's initial Fast Break week gave her the forward motion that spurred her to continue with more healthy changes to her lifestyle. This momentum in turn creates more healthy activities, which yield many ongoing benefits—more energy, less stress, better mood, and more restful sleep.

Choosing Your Fast Break Goals

By starting modestly with a Fast Break, you get off on the right foot and achieve a small win on your way to many more. Fast Breaks should be small and simple.

Here are some examples of typical Fast Break combinations. You can eat four servings of complex carbs, do ten minutes of cardio exercise, and write in a journal. Or you can drink eight cups of water, walk 15 minutes, and talk to a supportive friend.

Here are some Fast Break goals from which to choose. Choose one goal from each category. Try to do the goals you choose at least five of the next seven days, or daily if you can.

Nutritional Goals	Fitness Goals	Motivational Goals
Eat a breakfast that's high in fiber and protein	Exercise for ten minutes	Tell one person about your goals
Eat two fruits or vegetables	Do something active outdoors	Give yourself a five-minute mental pep talk
Don't drink soda	Stretch for ten minutes	Post a message on Spark-People's message boards
Don't eat in front of the TV	Track calories burned	Read a motivational story or book
Pack your lunch	Work in the yard	Reward yourself
Drink eight cups of water each day	Do 15 minutes of exercise while watching TV	Read an inspirational quote
Eat some sort of fresh produce	Use a stress/squeeze ball	Listen to a get-up-and-go song every day

You may think, *But these goals are so small!*

But at SparkPeople, we want you to grow accustomed to something you may have never encountered before in any diet or self-improvement program—ease, pleasure, and success.

Here's member MEDIAROCKS:

> *The Fast Break goals gave me a place to start without overwhelming me. I started with water and moving around (exercise) in smaller increments and then increased them with time. This took the "overwhelm" out of changing my lifestyle and gave me the tools I needed to get to where I am now. I believe anyone can use these tools to better their lives.*

In sharp contrast to our Fast Break goals, other programs often encourage monumental moves. They ask that you lose 20 pounds in a month by cutting out all carbs, fats, and sugars, run several miles each day, and use willpower to deprive yourself whenever you're tempted.

According to a recent SparkPeople poll, most dieters lose momentum in two weeks. Five pounds down, then another three. Then gridlock. You've hit a plateau and are stalling out and about to give up—it's just all too much.

Momentum is one of the hardest things to maintain when you choose to diet. Our Fast Break goals are modest enough to allow you to stay focused and consistent for the first week, but still effective enough to impact weight loss, especially over the long term, in the following weeks. They provide a solid base by easing your body—and mind—into the routine of eating better, exercising regularly, and staying motivated, thus setting you up for future success. Meeting and tracking these goals each day builds the habit of achievement and begins to ingrain new habits into your lifestyle.

Thinking about one step at a time is not only helpful as you start out it's also a great philosophy to keep in mind throughout your entire journey. As these single steps accumulate, they add up to big changes. Like our member AMYSJOY tells us:

> I just keep saying, one more water, one more minute on the treadmill, one teeny little tiny minute for me . . . makes one more pound . . . and now that one pound is 36 pounds gone! Look at me now!

Or member JEEPFAN:

> I guess I started out just wanting to get the hang of things again and get some control. So my Fast Break goals were pretty simple: get some type of exercise in daily—at that point anything; drink enough fluids—cutting out the soda; track everything I did—so I would have a better picture of my issues. Well, it worked; in the first two weeks I lost 10 pounds. . . . I have more endurance because I got to the exercising part. I have more strength. I eat better. And I am starting to sleep more again. Yeah! I guess I could say the Fast Break goals started me along a really positive path.

Action Step: Write down your three Fast Break goals here:

1.

2.

3.

PLAN YOUR SPARKTIME

We designed the SparkPeople program to fit your life, but you still need to plan ahead so you know where to find the time each day to make this work.

We recommend that you schedule ahead of time to:

- *Plan and review:* this could be five to ten minutes, either in the morning to plan for the day ahead or in the evening to plan the following day

- *Read and reflect:* build in time for short activities that serve your Fast Break goals, such as reading an inspirational story or telling your goals to a friend

- *Exercise:* our program is designed around ten-minute chunks of exercise that easily fit in your day

If you can figure out now how to shift other things around, then you'll be ready for success each day. Try to get your family's or friends' support for taking this time for yourself if necessary. They might even be able to join in some of your action steps.

By planning now, you'll be ready to shout to the world: "It's my SparkTime!"

Action Step: Choose a time each day to review and plan. Set up an electronic calendar or invest in a small desk calendar that will be dedicated to these changes you're making in your healthy lifestyle. Write down your plan!

REAFFIRM YOUR FOCUS

What's on your mind right this minute? Probably dozens of disconnected strands of obligation, duty, and daily concerns—your latest deadline for work, the time of your daughter's swim meet, your husband's bonus, or a homework assignment due at the end of the week. Your personal goals may be hovering somewhere in your consciousness, but they're probably far down the list.

But your Fast Break week is the time to reorganize your mind so that your goals are front and center, at the top of the hierarchy.

Earlier in the book, you read about setting goals and the importance of focus in making long-lasting changes in your life. Having specific, meaningful goals provides a guiding light that keeps you moving forward, infusing your daily activities and decisions with meaning. Now it's time to reaffirm the goals you set in Chapter 2 and refocus on them. Or, if you haven't yet considered your goals, it's time to set them now.

If you didn't set a long-term goal in Part I, please do so now. Concentrate on your long-term goals—and even your purpose and values, if you know those at this point. We'll use the Fast Break to help you practice setting and completing short-term action steps to move toward these long-term goals. The reason to write them down now is so that we can help you use them for incredible motivation as you make your healthy lifestyle change.

Once you've put your goals on paper, every time you are faced with a choice during your healthy lifestyle adventure—whenever you are confronted with a desire to forego your exercise or head back to the drive-thru for fried chicken and biscuits—you'll be able to visualize your goals or actually look at them. Simply thinking about your goals before you make a choice will increase the odds that you'll make a healthy, positive choice. You'll be able to say to yourself: *Here's what I want and why.*

If you've already written down your goals, take a moment to remind yourself why you chose them in the first place and why they're important.

For Sue, her goal wasn't simply losing 50 pounds. Her larger goals were to be involved again in meaningful work she loved and to be fit and active in the world.

Another member, CPCJONES01, recently sent me this note about her reasons for getting healthy:

> *No words can express my gratitude. I have only been a member for a short time but the difference it has made in my life and attitude toward healthy eating and exercise has changed dramatically for the good. I always thought I couldn't lose weight or that I was too far gone/too old to exercise. However, I now know that I CAN turn my life around for the better. You see, I have two grown daughters, and I am their only parent—that is the reason I want to get healthy and be around for them as long as possible. Thank you from the bottom of my heart.*

What about you? Do you want to lose ten pounds to help ease the arthritis in your hips? To be a positive role model for your child? To be able to run a marathon?

If you haven't come up with your goals yet, consider the following questions. What's important to you? What are your core beliefs? What truly drives you? What is your purpose in life? Is there a clash between what you really believe and what you're trying to accomplish?

Now think about your specific goals. What do you want to accomplish? Remember that your goals should be:

- *Unique:* based on your own dreams and life experience

- *Concrete:* exact and time-specific, such as "I want to run a 5K in three months" (just remember to give yourself some flexibility with exact weight-loss goals)

- *Inner-directed:* based on your own unique and specific reasons—"I want to lose five pounds in order to be able to walk up the stairs without losing my breath"

- *Harmonious:* in tune with your deep beliefs

- *Realistic:* challenging without being overwhelming—losing 40 pounds in one month is not possible without going on an extreme diet

- *Written:* so that you can see what you're working toward—writing the words five pounds in four weeks puts it into black and white and keeps it in your consciousness

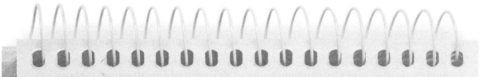

Action Step: Write your goals down as clearly as possible so you can refer back to them whenever you need a little motivation. (*My goals are to . . .*) Next, divide your goals into three categories: long-term goals (usually one year or more, but can be shorter depending on the goal), medium-term milestones (usually one to three months), and short-term action steps (usually one month or less).

Make a Vision Collage and Goal Reminders

Sue made several vision collages that reminded her why she wanted to become healthy and fit again. She found earlier photos of herself when she was working with children, as well as pictures of her riding the bicycle that had been sitting in her garage now for years. She found magazine photos of friends interacting with each other, and she cut out beach and mountain scenes of places she'd always wanted to travel. When she grew discouraged, she went and looked at these images hanging in her study or by her bedroom mirror, a spot where she often felt despondent. Instead of vague wishes, these were concrete, positive reminders of the goals she could reach if she persevered and remained motivated.

Action Step: If you haven't made the vision collage that we discussed in Part I, please do this now. Place it somewhere you can see it daily at a glance—not inside a desk drawer. I placed my vision collage on the wall in my office.

When life gets busy, hectic, and stressful, it's easy to forget your goals. But your vision collage will quickly help remind you of what's most important. This powerful tactic takes only a few seconds but has the potential to turn your whole day around or help you make a positive decision.

You can place other goal reminders in strategic areas too. Put them anywhere they'll help you—places where you spend the most time, such as your car, office, or computer area. And remember to post them in locations where you often lose your resolve. If you want to get healthier to stay active with your kids, you might find a picture of yourself playing with your kids and post it on your refrigerator or the pantry door.

Our goal is to surround your entire life with the motivation you need to succeed—this is just one small part of that goal!

SET UP SHOP

You're on the highway headed to an out-of-town conference and all of a sudden you feel your blood sugar drop.

You only grabbed a coffee and pastry for breakfast, and now you're paying the price, heading for an important meeting feeling shaky and weak. The only edible item in your glove compartment is a dried-up nutrition bar, circa 2005. You don't have many options on the interstate, and you need something filling and fast. You need gas anyway, so you stop at a convenience store and drive the rest of the way drinking a soda and ripping open bags of salty treats.

This is where planning ahead and setting up shop comes in.

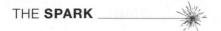

Your shop is wherever you spend your time—your house, your job, even your car. If your cupboards are full of cookies, your refrigerators stocked with sugary sodas, and your gym clothes hidden somewhere in the bottom of your closet, you won't be prepared to get started on your weight-loss and fitness goals. Millions of people hope to lose weight, yet only a few actually prepare for it. The rest treat it like a treasure hunt, setting off on a quest, ambling around, searching under this rock or that, hoping they'll find their way as they go.

Let's do it differently this time by setting up solid preparations that will be there, in place, when you are ready to go. In this way, you're acting as your own forward scout, paving the way for success.

As member HONEYLEA, co-leader of SparkPeople's 100 Plus First Step Club, says:

> *You have to make the commitment of time and effort. Losing weight is not something that will happen because you wish it to be so.*

Here are some strategies you can use right now to be more prepared. But remember, you don't have to do all of this at once. Start where you feel it will have the most impact, and then proceed from there.

Take a "Before" Photo

Any journey is more meaningful when you have a memento commemorating the place from which you first embarked. Even if you don't like looking at photos of yourself at the moment, consider taking one so that you can chronicle your success along the way.

Many SparkPeople members are motivated by these "before" photos. Once they make a healthy lifestyle change, lose weight, and become more active, they add an "after" photo, showing themselves finishing a race or posing in old clothes. These photos become a valuable reminder of how far they've traveled and are a crucial part of keeping track of their journey.

Prevent Temptations

Restock your kitchen. Do a full kitchen inspection. Begin replacing unhealthy foods with healthier alternatives. Don't worry if you can't accomplish this all at once. Just target a few strategic areas. This is a flexible process, so start where you feel comfortable and progress with time and practice.

- Stock up on whole-grain bread, pasta, and crackers.

- Buy fresh fruits and veggies. To make them even more accessible, buy them already washed and cut up if you don't want to spend time in preparation. Canned and frozen varieties are also nutritious and take less time.

- Get rid of sugary sodas.

- Make sure you have plenty of water—and a reusable water bottle for home, work, and your car.

- Banish junk food with empty calories; replace potato chips and cookies with energy-boosting granola bars, fruit, low-fat popcorn, or low-fat yogurt.

- Replace high fat with low fat. Low-fat cheeses, milks, and yogurts can make a big difference in calories.

Take Healthy Snacks to Work

Pack nutritious and filling apples, bananas, and almonds and keep them in your office. When the munchies come calling, you won't run to the vending machine and succumb to a candy bar.

Our member Chasity, who lost 111 pounds on SparkPeople, found success by making small changes that helped her succeed:

> I had no idea how much I was eating, how often I was eating, or even what I was actually eating. Adding things to the Nutrition Tracker forced me to be accountable for what I was consuming, and it made me think about the ingredients of the things I was eating. When I changed my eating habits, everyone around me noticed—and many of them changed theirs, too! My office became a much healthier place—we traded five-pound bags of M&M's for one-pound bags of raw, unsalted almonds!

Stock Healthy Snacks at Home

You've got a 7:00 date at an Italian restaurant, and you've been starving yourself all day so that you can eat what you want. By the time you reach the restaurant, you're so hungry that you fall on the bread-and-butter basket, order a fatty appetizer, and don't slow down until after dessert. Rather than depriving yourself this way, stock healthy snacks at home. Have a glass of vegetable juice, a small handful of almonds (protein and fat keep you full), low-fat cheese on a couple whole-grain crackers, or a tangerine before you leave—these will keep you sated and less desperate to fill up once dinnertime comes around. Though it seems counterintuitive, eating a light snack before you go out will allow you to savor your meal and all of its delicious flavors.

Make It Easy to Get Moving

It's hard to keep your commitment to exercise when getting ready to work out is a major production. You can make it easier by making sure the gear you need is on hand.

Pack a gym bag and keep it in your car for use on a moment's notice. Keeping these items handy makes it more likely that you'll follow your fitness impulse rather than heading home to your couch.

Walking is the cheapest and easiest form of exercise, but to walk comfortably you shouldn't wear your high heels, your work shoes, or your floppy sandals. The most important piece of fitness equipment you'll need is a good, comfortable pair of workout shoes. Make sure you have the right pair of sturdy shoes at the ready.

If you want to work out at home, shop wisely. Big equipment purchases aren't necessary. Start with some home-gym basics (exercise ball, resistance band, jump rope, small dumbbells) and build over time. No need for a trendy, expensive gym membership if the local fitness center has what you'll actually use or you're set up to get enough exercise at home. In fact, establishing a standard at-home exercise routine will prevent you from skipping out of your daily workout if you can't get to the gym on certain days.

Action Step: Choose some or all of these strategies to set up shop, and set yourself up for success.

CHOOSE YOUR REWARDS

You may be accustomed to diet-plan punishments—restrictions, deletions, and banishments. But at SparkPeople we don't believe in punishment, we believe in reward. Rewards are great motivators that can help you push forward to the finish line. Making a healthy lifestyle change is so important for the rest of your life that you deserve a reward for making it happen.

Many people approach changing their health habits from a position of pain. They berate themselves for their bad habits and expect nothing less than perfection in their efforts to change. But rewards and positive feedback are far more effective than punishment and criticism.

Imagine working for a boss who notices every single mistake you make, reminds you of these mistakes at every opportunity, belittles you, points out your faults, minimizes achievement whenever you start to feel good about yourself, never acknowledges what you do right with so much as a kind word or small reward . . . That's a strange way to motivate people! Yet that's exactly what we often do to ourselves when dieting. And then we wonder why our motivation disappears.

Let's try another approach. Find ways to use regular rewards to boost your morale. Instead of paying attention to what you do wrong, try focusing more on what you do right.

Make sure you accept that you deserve rewards. Negative self-talk may have you convinced that you haven't done anything special enough to earn them. That's the old, ineffective "boss" talking. Give yourself permission to be a good, supportive boss, and you'll get the personal performance you're looking for.

Action Step: For this action step, you should choose two rewards. First, select a small reward for completing all of your Fast Break goals on at least five of seven days. Second, select a larger reward for making it through all four stages. These rewards can be anything—from buying yourself some flowers to giving yourself some downtime to purchasing a new workout shirt. If you'd like some help selecting a reward, turn to the "Reward Yourself" section in Chapter 8. Now, write these rewards down next to your goals so you can use them for motivation.

LEARN WHAT YOU EAT

If you laid out on a picnic table everything you ate in a given day, you might find the display surprising. Did you really consume that half bag of potato chips, that mound of lasagna, that whole pile of cookies?

Eating, like breathing, is an act that most of us aren't conscious of as we rush through our days. We grow hungry—or frustrated or lonely—and we find something that fills us up or makes us feel temporarily better. It's often a blur of grabbing a bite, grazing off our child's plate in between deadlines, gobbling a meal on the run. Yet the quality and quantity of our food intake often elude us.

For the last three days of this first week, we'd like you to begin focusing on what you're eating—simply becoming aware of what would be arranged on that picnic table at the end of each day. We're not going to ask you to alter what you're consuming, or to worry about it—just begin to be conscious of it.

Track Your Food

Members are often surprised by how much they've been eating once they track their food. And they're often confused by portion size. Of all successful members, 65 percent measure their portions before they eat.

It's easy to fudge the truth when you're not paying attention. That Cobb salad drenched with oily dressing and fried chicken is mentally filed as a "vegetable" and transformed into a healthy lunch. In memory, four pieces of pizza metamorphose magically into one. Grazing directly from the refrigerator or off the stovetop doesn't even count.

Once members begin tracking their food, they're often shocked to learn that they're eating the equivalent of 4,000 calories a day, or that some of their favorite foods are actually calorie culprits. Others experience a sort of "perception gap" where they honestly believe they are drinking enough water or eating enough protein, only to learn after tracking that they really aren't.

Once you start logging your food intake, you'll see how awareness is in itself a huge step that will change the way you look at what you put into your body each day. That's what our community team member RAINY found:

> When I started, I . . . concentrated on building some awareness of what I was eating by consistently logging what I'd had and by establishing a loosely scheduled time to eat, rather than just grazing all day. [I learned that] I wasn't just grazing; I was eating the equivalent of six or more full meals a day!

Action Step: Start from where you are. If you've started a journal as we suggested in Chapter 4, you can carry that with you at all times and use it to log your food. Or copy the trackers in Appendix G of this book, or go to SparkPeople.com/myspark/nutrition.asp to track online. Next, write down each time you eat or drink something, no matter how small. If it goes into your mouth, it should go into your notebook. Write down what you ate, how much of it you ate, and how many calories it contained. Most food labels give you all the necessary information you need, for foods or recipes without labels, you can use the free online calorie counter at SparkPeople.com. Or, there are dozens of calorie counting books sold at bookstores.

That's all we want you to do—note it; don't change it. No pressure, no guilt, no discouragement from sky-high expectations. Just simple awareness.

Once you've logged your food for three days, it's time to take stock, to look back at your food log so that you can learn how, why, and when you eat.

What You Eat and How Much

It's easy to guesstimate what you're eating until you actually see it written down in black and white. Then you come face to face with the facts—that what you may have perceived as a single serving of mashed potatoes was actually a triple-serving mound, or that the burger you thought was modest was actually a super-sized protein portion, enough for several days. And that all those bites out of the refrigerator, stolen snacks, and midnight nibbling you barely noticed could add up to enough calories for several meals.

Ask yourself:

- How many calories are you eating? Is it generally the same each day? If not, why?

- Are your meals well balanced, with adequate fruits and vegetables?

- Do you load most of your calories in one meal?

- Are you aware of portion sizes? In this era of exploding super-sized meals, it's easy to underestimate that large milkshake or that 16-ounce steak.

- Do you have a tendency to eat convenience foods and snacks?

- Do you drink water with your meals, or high-calorie sodas and fruit drinks?

- Do you count condiments? How often do you bathe healthy choices with fatty additions—a salad with blue-cheese dressing, a turkey sandwich with high-fat mayonnaise, air-popped popcorn with melted butter?

When and Where You Eat

- Do you eat breakfast?

- Are you a solitary eater, apt to binge when you're alone?

- Are you a social eater, liable to lose control when you're at a party or out with friends?

95

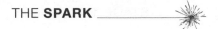

- Do you favor buffets or all-you-can-eat restaurants where the food just keeps on coming?

- Are you a drive-thru, fast-food cruiser?

- Do you tend to overeat when you're drinking alcohol?

- Do you tend to eat heavy dinners but skimp on breakfast and lunch?

- Do you graze all day without even realizing it?

- Does the routine of a workday keep you in line, while the freedom of the weekend weakens your willpower?

What's Your Mood While You're Eating?

Be aware of whether you're eating because you're really hungry or for emotional reasons.

- Is food a comfort when you're sad or lonely?
- Do you tend to eat when you're angry or disappointed?
- Does being overworked or under stress make you eat more?

What Are Your Triggers?

For Sue, the culprit was chocolate. When she felt lonely or discouraged, she headed to the kitchen cupboard and her stash of dark chocolate bars. Those first few bites of chocolate gave her a surge of comfort. The problem was that after one bite, she found herself unable to stop. Ten minutes later she'd be left with two or three empty wrappers and the feeling that she'd lost control.

Let's face it—there are certain foods and situations that bring out the worst in us and our eating habits. While it's true that five potato chips aren't a significant calorie load, you probably can't stop at five. Locate your own unique triggers—foods that make you lose control and simply want more. Common trigger foods are bread, ice cream, candy, chocolate, and salty snacks.

Don't beat yourself up about your results these first few days. Keeping track of typical days of food choices simply provides you with a better handle on what you need to work on—problem times, situations, or circumstances that make it difficult to eat healthfully.

CHAPTER 7

STAGE 2: HEALTHY DIET HABITS

So often people come to SparkPeople knowing that they want or need to lose weight but are unsure of how to do it. They're not certain what *really* works or which steps to take to get started. They often feel overwhelmed into inaction. They may want to go from "couch potato" to "everyday athlete," but they aren't sure how to get into the game and feel far from equipped to play.

That's where SparkPeople comes in. In this week, SparkPeople will become your coach, teaching you nutrition and exercise concepts that we've learned and developed over the past ten years. We'll teach you the basics that you need to know to get started and help you gain the skills you need that will act as your springboard to success.

With so much information out there, we want to give you the bottom line on what works, and keep it simple so you have the best shot at adopting these practices. The advice and strategies in this chapter are a combination of what has worked for tens of thousands of SparkPeople, what our coaches and experts know and see firsthand every day, and what the latest widely accepted scientific research tells us.

This week you'll learn new healthy habits—one at a time—that will easily fit into your lifestyle so that you will never need to diet again. At the same time, we'll continue weaving in strategies from each of the four cornerstones. It's time to use the hope and confidence you built in the Fast Break to start seeing even greater results. These next 7 days of our 28-day program will put you on that path!

WEEK 2 ACTION STEPS

This week we will focus on these action steps:

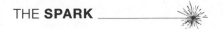

1. Take the Healthy Lifestyle Pledge
2. Adopt the top nutrition Secrets of Success
3. Track your food for weight loss following the SparkPeople nutrition guidelines
4. Exercise consistently ten minutes a day
5. Get adequate sleep

These action steps are simple, but there is magic in the combination. Sparking your-self in several areas at once leads to crisscross effects that create increased energy and motivation. And the power of consistent action is life-changing. Consistent action creates a power that multiplies as it grows. Looking ahead, after you learn the steps from this stage, stages 3 and 4 will do more than you can imagine to make this formula stick—in the form of a lasting healthy lifestyle.

THE HEALTHY LIFESTYLE PLEDGE

One of the best ways to reach a goal is to make a strong commitment to yourself. After reaching your Fast Break goals, you are now ready to take this to the next level.

Do you want to live a healthy lifestyle? Imagine for a moment what your life will be like when this happens. Visualize how it will feel to swim a lap, climb a hill, run a race. See yourself walking to class, playing ball with your kids, or doing a task as simple as climbing your stairs with grace and ease.

Are you ready to attain this fit and healthy body? If your answer is "YES!" then take our simple Healthy Lifestyle Pledge.

Action Step: Simply go to Appendix D in this book and sign your name to the Healthy Lifestyle Pledge. For even greater impact, tear out this page and keep it somewhere you'll see it regularly.

NUTRITION BASICS

When you sit down for dinner, you're not simply consuming a fat, a protein, and a starch. You're eating chicken, rice, and vegetables, which are composed of various amounts of these different nutrients—and more. Eating well is a result of consuming a balance of these nutritional elements. Understanding the makeup of the food you eat, your own optimal calorie range, and how to plan a meal are important basics we will introduce to you here.

Our goal is to empower you with knowledge. We're not simply showing you how to calculate your calorie range or plan a meal, but providing you with the skills you need to build a healthy lifestyle yourself. Our SparkPeople members tell us that this knowledge is a key motivator that sets them free to finally take control of their lives. Take our member LYNWAT, who lost 95 pounds and has maintained that weight loss for almost a year:

> *SparkPeople was such a big part of my success. I followed the advice that SparkPeople gives on calorie ranges and exercise. I log on every day and read articles . . . I have changed my eating habits and learned portion control. I still eat what I want, just less of it. I have also incorporated exercise into my daily life and I really enjoy it. SparkPeople helped me to get healthy and changed my life.*

What to Eat for Health

It's day one of your new way of eating. So what foods should you consume? With so many conflicting diet and nutrition messages out there, it can be confusing. We're so accustomed to hearing about fads and tricks that we've lost touch with the basic facts on what we should eat to lose weight. What you consume really does impact how your body functions, and deprivation diets do just that—deprive you of vital nutrients that keep you balanced and alive.

The food you eat is the source of energy and nutrition for your body, the fuel that allows you to get up in the morning, to run a marathon, and to bound up a flight of stairs at work. But you only have to gaze at the faces at a family banquet or join in a festive country potluck to know that food is not simply fuel, but also a source of pleasure. Your diet should be filled with food you enjoy, not food you see as a source of guilt or remorse.

Getting enough food may not be a problem, but obtaining good nutrition can be a challenge. What should you eat to stay healthy? Nearly everyone has an opinion, from your best friend to the morning newscaster, but the basics for good health haven't changed since the first fad diets were introduced. For optimum health, we recommend a balanced diet filled with a variety of good, whole foods that will contribute the over 45 different nutrients that your body needs each day. These can be divided into two classes: macronutrients (carbohydrates, proteins, and fat) and micronutrients (minerals such as iron, calcium, and zinc and vitamins such as vitamins A, B-12, and D).

Each nutrient has a particular job to perform in the building, maintenance, and operation of your body. Some jobs require that nutrients work together as a team. These jobs are nutrient-specific and cannot be done by other nutrients; an extra supply of one nutrient cannot make up for a shortage of another. That's why a balanced diet that includes a variety of foods from all food groups is so essential. Your body requires *all* these nutrients, not simply a few. Some must be replenished every day from food, while others can be stored in the body for future use.

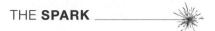

To eat a healthy, nutrient-packed diet, choose a wide variety of foods using these guidelines:

Choose Often (daily)	Limit (no more than 3–4 times/week)	Avoid (special occasions only)
Meat and Protein 2–4 servings/day		
Lean cuts of beef and pork (fat trimmed off), poultry (chicken and turkey) without skin, dried beans and peas, lentils, tofu, egg whites, egg substitutes, fish and shellfish, tuna canned with water	Egg yolks, fish sticks, tuna canned in oil, poultry with skin, chicken nuggets, turkey hot dogs, turkey bologna, nuts, peanut butter	Prime-grade meats, duck, goose, dark poultry meat, bacon, sausage, bologna, salami, hot dogs, ribs, organ meats, fried meats
Dairy and Calcium-rich Foods 2–3 servings/day		
Skim milk, 1% milk, 1% buttermilk, nonfat yogurt, nonfat frozen yogurt, fat-free cheese, low-fat cottage cheese, soy milk, soy cheese, other dairy-free milk substitutes	2% milk, 4% cottage cheese, ice milk, light cream cheese, light sour cream, low-fat yogurt, sherbet, low-fat cheese	Whole milk, regular cheese, cream, half-and-half, most nondairy creamers, real and nondairy whipped cream, cream cheese, sour cream, ice cream, custard-style yogurt
Fruits and Vegetables 5–9 servings/day		
Fresh, frozen, canned, or dried fruits and vegetables of all kinds	Olives, avocados, coconut	Fruits and vegetables prepared in butter or cream sauce, fried fruits and vegetables, vegetables with high-fat salad dressing
Grains 6–11 servings/day		
100% whole-grain breads, bagels, pasta, and cereals; oats; brown rice; bulgur; baked corn tortillas; low-fat crackers; air-popped popcorn; sprouted-grain bread; quinoa	White-flour breads; bagels; pasta; and cereals; angel-food cake; crackers; fat-free cakes and cookies; biscuits; fig bars; oatmeal-raisin cookies; pancakes; waffles; packaged mixes; white rice; granola	Croissants; pastry; pies; doughnuts; sweet rolls; snack crackers (with trans fats); grain products prepared with cream, butter, or cheese sauce
Fats and Oils 1–3 servings/day		
Olive oil, canola oil, peanut oil	Safflower, corn, soybean, sesame, sunflower oils, margarine, mayonnaise, lower-fat salad dressings, margarine that does not contain hydrogenated oil	Butter; lard; beef tallow; bacon fat; shortening; palm, palm kernel, and coconut oils; margarine or shortening made with hydrogenated oil

We also love the idea of adding "superfoods" to your diet—those foods that pack a powerful nutrient punch, foods like berries, spinach, and certain beans and grains. (For a full list of these foods, see the SparkPeople Website or Appendix B.)

The Balancing Act

Our ancestors would probably be amused by the hot debates over food in recent years—whether carbs, fats, or proteins are most important for health and optimal weight, and which should be stressed or ignored. When did eating become such a hotly contested topic, so complicated and controversial?

It shouldn't be. The truth is that generally accepted ranges were established for carbohydrates, fat, and protein intake after years of research that examined the relationship between nutrient intake and disease prevention. We believe these healthy ranges also help to ensure that a person is receiving a sufficient intake of other essential nutrients, vitamins, and minerals. The recommendations from the National Academy of Sciences are:

- 45 to 65 percent of calories eaten should come from carbohydrates.
- 20 to 35 percent of calories eaten should come from fat.
- 10 to 35 percent of calories eaten should come from protein.[1]

(Note: Because our members are striving to meet weight-loss goals through calorie restriction, we also recommend a minimum level of protein—at least 60 grams daily for women and 75 grams daily for men—to promote feelings of fullness and help prevent muscle loss.)

The SparkDiet takes a middle-of-the-road approach with these ranges. Our specific breakdown is approximately 50 percent carbohydrates, 30 percent fat, and 20 percent protein, all of which fall into the healthy ranges above. The table below converts The National Academy of Science's percentages into grams needed each day based on overall calorie intake:

Nutrient Healthy Range	Carbohydrates 45%–65%	Fat 20%–35%	Protein (Women) 10%–35%	Protein (Men) 10%–35%
1200 calories	135–195 g	27–47 g	60–105 g	N/A
1500 calories	169–244 g	33–58 g	60–131 g	75–131 g
1800 calories	203–293 g	40–70 g	60–158 g	75–158 g
2100 calories	236–341 g	47–82 g	60–184 g	75–184 g
2400 calories	270–390 g	53–93 g	60–210 g	75–210 g

Remember that your actual intake of carbohydrates, fat, and protein may be somewhat higher or lower than this, because of your taste preferences, cooking style, culture, fitness routine, health conditions, and day-to-day changes in diet. Do your best to meet at least the minimum recommendations.

All this may seem like a lot of information to "digest" and put into practice. But once you get started, you'll find that healthy eating really involves a natural, commonsense approach—real foods in sensible portions, the way your grandparents probably ate before the era of super-size drive-thrus—sitting down to a chicken breast, a nice portion of vegetables, a small starch, and a fresh piece of fruit.

We also believe in flexibility. This is your *life,* not a highly regimented military operation. At least 80 percent of the time, 96 percent of successful members eat a healthy diet. The majority (70 percent) don't cut out "bad foods." These successful members know something important: there is no such thing as perfection when it comes to dieting. They know that they will have indulgences and "imperfect" food days, and they build them into their plans. More importantly, they don't beat themselves up for it—if you do, it's a sure way to derail your efforts. It makes sense that when successful members have a bad food day, they don't worry about it because they eat healthy and exercise most of the time.

We strongly believe that to successfully build a healthy lifestyle and stick to it for the rest of your life, you need a philosophy that allows some flexibility and doesn't expect that you will never veer off track. In contrast to other programs that expect perfection, focus on deprivation, and set you up for long-term failure and disappointment, SparkPeople's plan fits into your real life and allows you to enjoy food without feeling guilty.

So relax and take it one step, one habit, even one meal at a time. It really does become easier with practice. One day it just "clicks," and the knowledge you've gained and the habits you've practiced become a seamless part of your new, healthier life.

This is what our member BERNADETTEA36, who has lost 50 pounds, discovered:

> *I used to rely on vitamins or bars to get my "nutrition." Now I know that you need proteins, whole grains, and veggies/fruits with every meal to make it balanced. I am now getting the right amounts. It feels great that I am on the right track! I know that I can continue with this lifestyle because I enjoy it and it has become part of who I am.*

BUILD YOUR OWN HEALTHY MEAL PLAN

We appreciate the individuality of our members, and we know that different people plan their meals differently. That's why we leave the way you build your meal plans up to you. Our Secrets of Success survey found that only a slightly higher percentage of successful people chose their own foods as opposed to those who followed structured meal plans, so it is an individual preference.

You can choose from:

- Your own daily diets based on the guidelines provided here

- Structured food plans generated for you at SparkPeople.com; you can use our online meal plans as is, or make substitutions based on seasonal foods, budget, and food preferences

- Other healthy eating plans that tell you what to eat at each meal, as long as they offer a balanced diet and they don't suggest severe calorie restriction; your health-care provider or a registered dietitian can provide you with a meal plan for your calorie range, too

Structured diets that take the guesswork out of what to eat make it easier for some people, while having the freedom of choice works better for others who feel deprived when they aren't choosing their own foods. Members have found success using both methods.

Any eating plan you choose should not make you feel deprived, but full, satisfied, and nourished. If you follow these guidelines, that's exactly how you *will* feel! And along the way, you'll discover how great healthy food can really taste.

Eating Strategies for Health and Weight Loss

Keep these strategies in mind when you're planning when, where, and what to eat throughout the day:

- Eat three meals daily and one or two planned snacks, keeping in mind your total calorie range.

- Plan to eat approximately the same number of calories at each meal throughout the day, with slightly more at breakfast and lunch. The total should be within your calorie range.

- Include approximately 15 to 20 grams of protein with each meal and 5 to 10 grams during each snack to promote fullness.

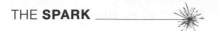

- To help with satiety, avoid eating carbohydrates without protein.

- Include a small amount of healthy fat at every meal; olive oil, nuts, seeds, flaxseed, peanut butter, and avocados all contain heart-healthy fats.

- Eat plenty of high-fiber food daily, aiming for 25 to 35 grams by the end of the day. Fiber comes from plant foods such as fruits (especially those with peels), vegetables, whole grains (brown rice, whole-wheat bread and cereals, oats), nuts, and seeds.

- Drink plenty of water; aim for eight cups a day.

- Have some protein and healthy fat, plus fiber, with every meal, to provide satiety as well as slow the time it takes your stomach to empty—making it longer until hunger strikes next.

- Drink water or a low-calorie beverage with your meals and in the evening.

- Don't eat mindlessly! Eat all meals and snacks at the table, keeping all of your attention on the food you're enjoying. Take your time and really enjoy every bite.

- Cook at home—77 percent of successful members proactively did more cooking at home to reach their weight-loss goals. It's the easiest way to control your portions, and it allows you to use more nutritious, lower-calorie alternatives in your preparations.

The Perfect Plate

You can use these guidelines as you're planning individual meals. The plate system is one way to put them into practice; it lets you build a healthy diet one meal at a time.

Think of your plate as a daily creation of nutrition and pleasure. Then perform the following review of your plate each mealtime to be certain it contains the following portions of different food types:

- Fill about one-quarter of your plate with starches such as brown rice, whole-wheat pasta, oats, whole-grain cereal, whole-wheat bread (two slices), potatoes, corn, or peas. Choose whole-grain carbohydrates whenever possible.

- Another quarter of your plate contain lean protein such as chicken, fish, meat, eggs, beans, and tofu.

- One-half of your plate should contain non-starchy vegetables like broccoli, carrots, cucumbers, lettuce, tomatoes, or cauliflower. For breakfast, include a generous portion of fruit instead of vegetables, such as berries, a pear, an orange, or a banana.

- Finish off the meal with a glass of skim milk, yogurt, a small portion of nuts or seeds, a piece of fruit, or a small roll, depending what you're in the mood for and/or what will help you meet your nutrient targets for the day.

SparkPeople Mix-and-Match Meals

An easy and delicious way to help you create healthy, balanced meals that fit these guidelines is to use the SparkPeople Mix-and-Match Meal charts. This is a simple system for coming up with great recipe ideas that fit perfectly into your diet. You can choose ingredients from several preselected categories, and mix and match any of them to come up with great combinations. You can use these for any meal, including breakfast, salads and sandwiches, and dinners. Choose any combination of the listed ingredients, and you'll get an average of 300 to 400 calorie meals. (SparkPeople's Mix-and-Match Meal charts and other great ideas for planning delicious and healthy meals can be found in Appendix A of this book, as well as online at SparkPeople.com/mixmatch)

To see how these meal guidelines might look when you put them all together into a daily meal plan, you can refer to the sample menus in Appendix A.

TOP NUTRITION SECRETS OF SUCCESS

Surveying our members has provided us with a treasure trove of information about how they've achieved optimum weight loss and fitness. Here's the best nutrition advice taken from what worked best for our most successful members.

Eat More Fruits and Veggies

In our Secrets of Success survey, across all successful segments, including those who lost over 100 pounds and those who have met their weight-loss goals in general, the number-one nutritional strategy was to eat *more* fruits and vegetables. Of those who met their goals and are at their ideal weight, 90 percent now eat more fruits and veggies.

Vegetables and fruits are nutrient powerhouses that fill you up, give you energy, and are full of antioxidants that are vital for optimum health. Not only do they provide essential nutrients but they also help you feel fuller and crowd out other, less healthful food choices.

Even if you don't currently love fruits and vegetables, we'll show you easy ways to fit them into your menus. One strategy that might seem unrelated at first glance is to start or increase your exercise. What does that have to do with eating? Well, members often report that once they've begun exercising regularly and feeling healthier, they start to actually "crave" healthier foods, including fruits and vegetables!

Remember to include plenty of *raw* fruits and vegetables, too—they are especially nutritious and require lots of chewing, which slows down your eating process and allows you to recognize that you are full. If you eat too quickly, you often eat more than you need because you haven't had time to realize when you've *actually* eaten enough.

Don't be discouraged by the recommended five servings a day; one serving is less than what you might think. One serving equals:

- 1 medium piece of fruit

- ½ cup fruit (raw, canned, or frozen)

- ½ cup cooked vegetables (canned or frozen)

- 1 cup raw vegetables

- ¼ cup dried fruit

- 4–6 ounces of 100 percent juice (serving size depends on the type of juice, so read labels)

- ½ cup cooked peas or beans

Action Step: Set a goal of getting at least five servings of fruits and vegetables throughout the day.

TIPS AND TRICKS FOR EATING MORE FRUITS AND VEGGIES

- Add fruit to your cereal, oatmeal, waffles, pancakes, or yogurt at breakfast.

- Snack on raw vegetables or fruits instead of chips or pretzels. Keep a fresh bag of sugar snap peas, nuts, raisins, or carrot sticks in your car, your office, or your backpack.

- Drink 100 percent juice instead of addictive coffee, tea, or soda, but limit your juice intake to no more than one cup daily.

- Going out to lunch? Take a trip to the grocery salad bar. Use lots of dark green leaves and other vegetables instead of piling on eggs, bacon, and cheese.

- Add frozen veggies to any pasta dish. It's an easy way to get in another serving.

- Add your own beans and vegetables (tomatoes, spinach, peppers, cabbage) to canned and quick-serve soups.

- If you have pizza, load on extra veggies and pineapple instead of fatty meats and extra cheese. (Try whole-grain crusts and low-fat cheese to make it even healthier.)

- Try berries, melons, or dates for a naturally sweet dessert rather than the usual candy bar, cookie, or ice-cream sandwich.

- Frozen fruit and veggies, as well as canned, are nearly as healthy as the fresh stuff (often healthier when the fresh varieties are not in season), and they take only minutes to prepare. When buying canned fruit, look for unsweetened or sugar-free varieties; choose sodium-free or low-sodium canned vegetables. Canned fruits and vegetables can be rinsed and drained to remove excess sugar or sodium, too.

- Combine fruit with your main meal courses. Raisins, apples, and tangerine slices add sweet, crunchy variety to a salad. Apples complement pork, pineapple is great with fish, and orange slices are perfect with chicken.

- Savor a smoothie, made with any combination of fresh or frozen fruit, low-fat milk, yogurt, ice, and 100 percent juice.

- Call on comfort foods. Add broccoli to macaroni and cheese, berries to ice cream, and frozen peas to casseroles.

Eat Breakfast

If you've heard it once, you've heard it a million times: breakfast is the most important meal of the day. Why? Because you've just spent eight hours in virtual hibernation, without food or water. You're dehydrated, and your blood sugar is so low that you have little energy. And now it's time to get to work or hurry the kids off to school before your own eight-hour day. More than at any other point, you need nourishment. Right now.

Almost all successful SparkPeople and all 100-pound losers either eat a substantial breakfast (66 percent) and or eat some breakfast (25.5 percent) every day—so over 90 percent eat at least some breakfast every day. Less than 1 percent of successful members skip breakfast altogether.

While every meal matters, when it comes to nourishing your body, eating breakfast is particularly important in helping you lose weight. That's because those who skip this critical meal tend to snack on unhealthy, high-calorie food before lunch and throughout the day and end up eating more calories than if they'd begun with a good foundational morning meal. Breakfast eaters, on the other hand, typically cruise through the morning, brimming with energy. By the time they reach lunch, they're more likely to make a healthy choice that helps them stay on track because they're not feeling weak and depleted.

SparkPeople recommends a breakfast that includes a mix of quality carbohydrates, healthy protein, and healthy fat, along with some fruit or vegetables. The average calorie range might be somewhere between 300 and 400 calories.

Here are some of our favorite healthy breakfast ideas:

- Incorporate complex carbohydrates, such as whole-wheat toast and bagels. Spread peanut butter and raisins on top for added flavor.

- Bake bran muffins early in the week. Make sure they are reasonably sized— somewhere between mini-muffins and the commonly oversized versions often found at a bakery. Grab a muffin and a glass of milk to make a complete breakfast.

- Prepare a breakfast casserole the night before. Pop it in the microwave when you wake up and it will be ready to go when you are.

- Make whole-grain waffles Sunday morning and freeze the leftovers. You can pop 'em in the toaster for a homemade breakfast. Also, grocery stores sell frozen whole-grain selections. Top them with fruit and nuts for greater nutrition and filling power.

- Have you ever tried a tortilla for breakfast? Wrap up cold turkey and cheese, grab an apple, and you're on your way.

- Don't forget cold cereal. We're not talking about the kind covered with sugar, but the healthy variety. Items such as bran flakes and shredded wheat usually make good choices.

- Whole-egg or egg-white omelets with fresh or frozen veggies (carrots, broccoli, celery, peppers, onions, and even black beans) help you meet your quota for vegetables and protein.

- Make a shake or a smoothie. Blend fruit and low-fat yogurt and then drink it in the car. A side option is a small bag of finger foods, such as a mixture of granola and grapes.

- Eat oatmeal! In a recent SparkPeople survey, oatmeal was the number-one breakfast choice of SparkPeople!

Action Step: Eat a substantial breakfast each day.

Drink Water

Despite water's many benefits, it is one of the most neglected parts of our diet. Some of us can go an entire day without drinking a single cup. But at SparkPeople, we're obsessed with water—and with good reason! Not only does it replace sugary, high-calorie drinks, but it is critical to feeling full, having energy, and losing weight. Of successful members, 74.5 percent drink eight cups of water every day. Only around half of those with a "diet" mentality get enough water. Those who lost at least 100 pounds report drinking even more than eight cups a day.

So do you really need eight cups? Like most recommendations, it depends. Everyone's needs are different and dependent on several factors, including your weight, how much you exercise, how many water-rich foods you eat, the amount of muscle mass you have, and the weather (conditions such as heat and humidity). But eight cups a day is still a good goal for the average person. The best way to find out how much you need is to check the color of your urine. It should look like you squeezed a lemon in it. If it's much darker, try drinking a little more water.

Okay, you're thinking, this is great advice, but how can you easily increase your daily water consumption? We've heard thousands of members go from asking, "How

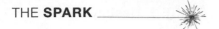

can I fit it in?" to saying, "I can't live without my eight cups a day!" Here are some great ways to get your daily water. Try the ones that appeal to you, and you'll see and feel the difference:

- Make your water bottle your constant companion.

- Fill your pitchers—leave full pitchers in the office or kitchen to remind you to drink throughout the day.

- Start your day with a big glass of water.

- Order water at restaurants instead of soda, tea, or a fruit drink.

- Flavor your water with citrus, cucumber, or flavored powders.

- Take more trips to the water cooler at work.

- Come up with a clever tracking system of your own—or track online at SparkPeople.com.

Action Step: Commit to drinking eight cups of water per day.

TRACK YOUR FOOD FOR WEIGHT LOSS

What you eat has everything to do with who you are. Not all five-foot-eight humans have the same calorie requirements. The variations between individual activity levels and lifestyles are enormous. That's why we encourage you to take the time to use our guidelines and come up with your own individual calorie consumption range.

Figuring out how much to eat is critically important. If your calorie consumption is too high, you'll obviously either gain or not lose weight, but it's equally important to not go too low, as this will also slow your progress.

So how do you figure out the right range? Both your food intake and your activity level affect your weight. Eating food provides your body with the energy it needs, while physical activity burns calories. So the key to successful weight loss seems simple—finding the right ways to balance the calories you consume with the calories you burn.

When you consume more calories than your body can use, the excess calories are stored as fat and you gain weight. To lose weight, you simply need to use more calories than you eat so your body is free to call upon other energy sources, such as stored fat.

Balancing the calories you consume with those you burn is the safest, healthiest way to manage your weight—for the next two weeks or the next 20 years. It takes about 3,500 calories to make one pound of fat. So to lose one pound, you can:

- Burn 3,500 excess calories through exercise alone (if you have a few hours to kill each day)

- Eat 3,500 fewer calories (starvation diet, anyone?)

- Combine exercise and calorie reduction (the best option)

For example, to lose one pound in a week, you could simply create a calorie deficit of 500 calories per day (7 x 500 = 3,500). This could be as simple as cutting out one donut (280 calories) and jogging for 25 minutes (240 calories) each day. As you've read already, there are also substantial crisscross effects between nutrition and fitness that go beyond numbers and make combining the two an even better choice.

How Many Calories Do I Need?

SparkPeople.com uses a ten-step formula to create a personalized calorie range for each person. We strongly encourage you to create your own free account at SparkPeople.com to get the most accurate calorie range for your goals. However, for the purposes of this book, you can use the simple charts below to estimate your body's calorie needs, based on your gender, current weight, and activity level. Please note the importance of being accurate and honest with yourself when selecting your activity level. Most people tend to overestimate how active they really are, but doing this could hurt your weight loss. When choosing your calorie needs based on your activity level, use these guidelines:

- *Little to no exercise.* You do not engage in planned fitness activities on a regular basis, but you may take part in some light physical activity through- out the day.

- *Light exercise.* You take part in planned workouts for up to 30 minutes a few times per week and/or spend two to three hours on your feet during the day.

- *Regular exercise.* You work out regularly and consistently for 30 to 60 min- utes, usually at a mild to moderate intensity, several times per week and spend two to three hours on your feet daily.

Find your daily calorie needs for weight maintenance on the charts below. These ranges are based on the Harris Benedict equation, which combines your basal metabolic rate (the number of calories you would burn in one day if you didn't move at all) and your activity level to determine how many calories you need to maintain your current weight. However, the ranges have been slightly adapted by SparkPeople Registered Dietitian Becky Hand.

DAILY CALORIE NEEDS FOR WEIGHT MAINTENANCE: FEMALES

Weight (lbs)	Little to no exercise	Light exercise	Regular exercise
110–120	1,600–1,625	1,700–1,725	1,850–1,875
121–130	1,626–1,650	1,726–1,750	1,876–1,900
131–140	1,651–1,675	1,751–1,775	1,901–1,925
141–150	1,676–1,700	1,776–1,800	1,926–1,950
151–160	1,701–1,725	1,801–1,825	1,951–1,975
161–170	1,726–1,750	1,826–1,850	1,976–2,000
171–180	1,751–1,775	1,851–1,875	2,001-2,025
181–190	1,776–1,800	1,876–1,900	2,126–2,150
191–200	1,801–1,825	1,901–1,925	2,151–2,175
201–210	1,826–1,850	1,926–1,950	2,076–2,100
211–220	1,851–1,875	1,951–1,975	2,101–2,125
221–230	1,876–1,900	1,976–2,000	2,126–2,150
231–240	1,901–1,925	2,001–2,025	2,151–2,175
241–250	1,926–1,950	2,026–2,050	2,176–2,200
251–260	1,951–1,975	2,051–2,075	2,201–2,225
261–270	1,976–2,000	2,076–2,100	2,226–2,250
271–280	2,001–2,025	2,101–2,125	2,251–2,275
281–290	2,026–2,050	2,126–2,150	2,276–2,300
291–300	2,051–2,075	2,151–2,175	2,301–2,325
301–310	2,076–2,100	2,176–2,200	2,326–2,350
311–320	2,101–2,125	2,201–2,225	2,351–2,375

DAILY CALORIE NEEDS FOR WEIGHT MAINTENANCE: MALES

Weight (lbs)	Little to no exercise	Some exercise	Regular exercise
121–130	1,700–1,750	1,956–2,010	2,301–2,360
131–140	1,751–1,800	2,011–2,065	2,361–2,420
141–150	1,801–1,850	2,066–2,120	2,421–2,480
151–160	1,851–1,900	2,121–2,175	2,581–2,540
161–170	1,901–1,950	2,176–2,230	2,541–2,600
171–180	1,951–2,000	2,231–2,285	2,601–2,660
181–190	2,001–2,050	2,286–2,340	2,661–2,720
191–200	2,051–2,100	2,341–2,395	2,721–2,780
201–210	2,101–2,150	2,396–2,450	2,781–2,840
211–220	2,151–2,200	2,451–2,505	2,841–2,900
221–230	2,201–2,250	2,506–2,560	2,901–2,960
231–240	2,251–2,300	2,561–2,615	2,961–3,020
241–250	2,301–2,350	2,616–2,670	3,021–3,080
251–260	2,351–2,400	2,671–2,725	3,081–3,140
261–270	2,401–2,450	2,726–2,780	3,141–3,200
271–280	2,451–2,500	2,781–2,835	3,201–3,260
281–290	2,501–2,550	2,836–2,890	3,261–3,320
291–300	2,551–2,600	2,891–2,945	3,321–3,380
301–310	2,601–2,650	2,946–3,000	3,381–3,440
311–320	2,651–2,700	3,001–3,055	3,441–3,500

People who weigh more than 320 pounds should create an account at SparkPeople.com for the utmost accuracy regarding their calorie needs. However, as a rough estimate, start with the appropriate column for your activity. Then, for each 10 pounds you weigh over 320 pounds, add 25 calories if you are female and 50 calories if you are male.

Planning to Lose

Now that you have your calorie range for weight maintenance, you can estimate how many calories you need to cut from your diet each day to reach your goal weight.

Using the numbers you found on the chart above, refer to the guidelines below to safely cut enough calories to lose up to one pound per week. If you want to lose up to two pounds per week, you need to do so by exercising to burn extra calories each day. The reason is that simply cutting enough calories to lose two pounds per week is not the best strategy—it can hurt your chances of making this a true lifestyle change compared to a typical "diet." Cutting even more calories to lose weight—instead of burning extra calories by exercising—can also result in hunger and make it harder for you to meet your body's needs for vitamins, minerals, and other nutrients.

If you are:

- Less than 25 pounds from your goal weight, subtract 200 calories from each end of your calorie range

- Between 26 and 50 pounds from your goal weight, subtract 350 calories from each end of your calorie range

- Between 51 and 100 pounds from your goal weight, subtract 500 calories from each end of your calorie range

If you are over 100 pounds from your goal weight, you can safely lose more than two pounds per week, up to one percent of your body weight per week. To get the most accurate calorie range for this level of weight loss, create an account at SparkPeople.com. For the purposes of this book, average your current weight and your goal weight, and then follow the calorie needs for maintaining that weight on the chart. (For example, a woman who weighs 400 pounds but wants to weigh 200 pounds would start out using the calorie range for 300 pounds to lose weight. Once she reaches 300 pounds, she is within 100 pounds of her goal weight. So, she should refer to the bullet points above, subtracting 500 calories from each end of the 300 pound calorie range in the chart.)

Remember to readjust your calorie intake with your weight loss. If you start needing to lose 50 pounds, subtract 350 calories from each end of your calorie range. However, once you are within 25 pounds of your goal weight, switch to the guidelines requiring that you subtract only 200 calories from each end.

Don't Cut Calories Too Far

People who want to lose weight quickly often begin by starving themselves, gritting their teeth, and setting the stage for deprivation: coffee for breakfast, yogurt for lunch, salad for dinner. Not only is this famine approach unhealthy, but just as importantly, it doesn't *work.* You can actually harm your ability to lose weight by falling too low in calorie intake. Your body has a protective mechanism: when it feels as if it's starving—if calories drop too low—your body tries to conserve energy and hold on to every precious fat cell. Going into such a "starvation mode" lowers metabolism, conserves calories and fat, and prevents you from losing weight.

For your health and safety, women should never eat fewer than 1,200 calories daily and men should never consume fewer than 1,500. If you did the math and came up with a range below this, round up. This minimum calorie level is one of the most important ways to make a healthy lifestyle change instead of continuing a diet mentality. By eating enough calories each day, you increase the odds that you will "stick" to your healthy goals and finally stay on an upward spiral. It's simple to see why: life isn't easy or fun when you are hungry, it's hard. When you are eating enough, it's easier to stay focused on your goals.

Weigh-In Guidelines

Our guidelines are to weigh in no more than once a week. When doing so, make sure to always weigh in under the same circumstances—at the same time of day, wearing comparable clothing, with or without eating or drinking water. First thing in the morning, before breakfast, is usually the best and easiest time.

In general, however, we recommend that people weigh in even less, such as once every two weeks or even once a month.

It's fine to weigh yourself as a way of keeping yourself accountable and of monitoring one aspect of your health. But try not to let that scale be your main motivator. No matter what little fluctuations you might see, notice overall trends: not hour-to-hour or day-to-day changes.

In order to stay motivated, find other ways to measure your progress instead of stepping on the scale. Try some of the following benchmarks that are much more meaningful and motivating:

- *Body measures:* clothing size; waist, hip, neck, and arm measurements; fitting into favorite clothes

- *Performance:* more endurance during exercise; being able to train harder, longer, or faster; playing a sport better

- *General feeling:* energy level, confidence, attitude, outlook, and thinking ability; how often you feel sleepy during the day

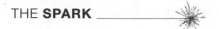

- *Health:* blood pressure, cholesterol level, blood sugar level

- *Intangibles:* how you look, compliments you receive, how others respond to you

Get Tracking!

By now you have grown accustomed to paying attention to what you eat—keeping track of the array of food on the virtual picnic table at the end of each day. We want you to continue tracking for the next three weeks—and beyond—but with a crucial difference. While before you tracked food in order to build awareness, now we want you to log what you're eating as a tool to planning your meals and staying within your recommended calorie range.

Over time, you may find you don't need to track everything, but when you make changes to your diet, tracking can remain a really helpful tool. In our Secrets of Success survey, we found that about half of successful members track their food every day, and most track their food either every day, several times a week, or periodically, as a tool to get them back on track.

At the end of the book, in Appendix G, you'll see food tracker pages that will help you log what you eat. There is also a fully interactive tracker online for members at SparkPeople.com/myspark/nutrition.asp. If you haven't joined the SparkPeople community, follow the link for the online book program at SparkPeople.com/TheSpark.

Action Step: Track your food five to seven days per week for the next three weeks. In addition to tracking to stay within recommended calorie/fat/protein/carbohydrate ranges, pay special attention to eating a substantial breakfast, trying to get five or more servings of fruits and vegetables in daily, and drinking eight or more cups of water. To see how all of this might come together in a daily menu plan, check out the sample menus in Appendix A.

EXERCISE CONSISTENTLY

One of our wise members once said that the difference between exercising and not exercising was the difference between waking and remaining asleep. Our bodies are meant for exercise and actually crave it. And exercise rapidly pays you back with increased feelings of stamina, strength, and well-being.

At SparkPeople we know that exercise is one of the most powerful aspects of a healthy lifestyle. Besides being a potent weight-loss tool, it is a real tonic for every aspect of your life—a booster of strength, health, and spirit that wakes you up and makes you feel more focused and alive.

The exercise section of the program is short for a crucial reason. Instead of overwhelming you with everything there is to know about exercise, we simply want you to learn one of the most powerful strategies in the entire SparkPeople program—that exercise done consistently will change your life, even if it is short workouts. In fact, at the beginning, short workouts are actually a better way to build this consistency.

For these three weeks, we're asking you to make the commitment to exercise every day (or at least five days a week). There is a reason we recommend you exercise every day, especially at this stage. Exercise is one of the most powerful elements of this program, given its ability to change your weight, mood, energy level, productivity level, and sleep, even what you can accomplish in your life. In order to switch from "trying to get around to fitting in exercise a few times a week" to making exercise an integral part of your life most days, you'll need to make sustained, consistent effort.

Action Step: For these next three weeks, we want you to commit to just ten minutes a day of some type of activity. Ideally, four of these days will be cardio, two strength training, and one either active recovery (light exercise) or a rest day. Just ten minutes a day! Appendix C in the back of the book includes several detailed ten-minute workouts.

Of course, if you are already someone who exercises and your workouts are longer than ten minutes, please continue. Or if you feel like doing more than ten minutes, that's also great as long as you exercise every day. In this stage, however, we're more interested in consistency than in long, vigorous workouts.

The purpose of the exercise guidelines in this book is to get you started and consistent—the most important part of an exercise program. Once you have mastered this, there are more detailed exercise plans in the online book program. Another option is the SparkPeople exercise DVD that can be used alongside this book.

The Magic of Ten Minutes

No matter how busy you are, you can carve out at least ten minutes in your day, right? That's all you need to initiate a simple exercise program that can eventually transform your life.

If finding the motivation to work out has been a daunting task, our ten-minute workouts are a great place to start. Even though ten minutes of exercise won't burn as many calories as an hour, it still burns calories, which is more than no exercise at all. Exercising consistently over time, even for shorter durations, burns more calories overall than bursts of vigorous activity followed by days of no activity, and it's certainly better for your overall health.

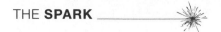

In addition to helping lay the foundation of a consistent exercise program, this ten-minute strategy also prevents you from stopping completely when time is tight. This is critical, as so many of us fall off the workout wagon because our expectations are too high.

These mini-workouts will help you turn exercise into a habit, not a special occasion or an all-or-nothing event. And after doing these ten-minute workouts consistently for a while, you'll begin to notice improvements that will motivate you to do even more—and your energy level will slowly start to increase. Regardless of your current level of activity, short workouts can be a great source of motivation and the "spark" you need to move your program into gear!

Ten-minute workouts can include easy exercises you can do at home, when you get up in the morning, or while you're making dinner or waiting for the laundry. Pick something you enjoy so you're more likely to stick with it.

Learning to Love Exercise

Do you feel a great internal groan at the thought of exercising every day? If so, take heart. Our members regularly tell us that once they begin to exercise, it transforms their lives, and they actually crave the energized, wide-awake feeling it gives them. In fact, one of the most striking results of our Secrets of Success survey is that successful members were less likely than "dieters" to view exercise as a chore. Of those who met their goals, only half of them actually liked exercise before they started SparkPeople, and 75 percent enjoy it now. And a full 96 percent either like it, love it, or at least love how it makes them feel when they're done! Take our member REVSERENA:

> I usually dread exercise before I start. Once I'm a few minutes in it starts to feel good. As I reach the end of my workout I almost always feel GREAT! Recognizing this pattern has really helped me overcome the inertia and reluctance that used to keep me on the couch. I exercise pretty vigorously most days now.

Our member DDOORN reminds us that exercise isn't only about going to the gym to burn calories, but also about expanding boundaries, having fun, and living life to the fullest.

> I am so proud of ALL the barriers which have been overcome as my fitness and health have improved over the last few years with the tremendous support of SparkPeople. Yesterday I tried cross country skiing for the first time EVER! A few years ago I couldn't even CONCEIVE of such an action! I'm riding my bicycle over 20 miles a trip . . . INCOMPREHENSIBLE to my

old, unhealthy self. On the treadmill, I find myself JOGGING through my favorite songs . . . I find myself increasingly addicted to new challenges . . . thinking about rollerblading/skating, biking longer distances, getting back into a canoe, taking dancing lessons . . . the sky's the limit! It's this feeling of physical freedom and unlimited potential that I am most proud of since reclaiming my fitness!

SLEEP WELL

Who would think that sleep—a passive activity that requires no motivation or effort—would be so essential to weight loss and maintaining a healthy lifestyle? Yet it is. Sleep has such amazing crisscross effects that it deserves a place as one of the most important elements of the program. The 28-day program is designed to be easy to follow, and good sleep makes it even easier.

Let's take a look at just a few ways that lower energy levels from lack of sleep can hold you back—and even lead you into a downward spiral:

- *Focus.* Poor sleep makes it more difficult to focus on taking small, consistent steps to reach your goals.

- *Exercise.* Ten minutes of fitness is easy. But when you're tired, even ten minutes becomes physically and mentally more difficult.

- *Motivation and support.* Without sleep, you become grumpy and impatient with yourself and others. This means you could lose two of your most important sources of support—positive pep talks from yourself and encouragement from friends and family.

- *Stress.* Poor sleep makes you sensitive to small issues. It also makes you more easily discouraged.

Among successful members and 100-pound losers, one of the most common healthy activities is getting enough sleep. In fact, increased sleep correlated with more weight loss across the board. Over 70 percent of 100-pound losers regularly get enough sleep, between seven to eight hours per night on average. Of those who reported being "stuck," unable to lose weight, and practicing a "diet" mentality, only about 50 percent got enough sleep, averaging five to seven hours a night.

Of course, looking at these statistics, it's hard to tell if sleep was a big factor in helping the members achieve their fitness and nutrition goals or if consistent exercise and better nutrition helped them get better sleep. But, from what we see among our successful members, it's probably a combination of these things that crisscross and create an upward spiral in which they feel better and improve in many aspects of their lives at the same time. This is a key to the SparkPeople program.

Here are some more sleep facts:

- Burning the midnight oil could give you the munchies the next day. In a small study, 12 young men slept for only four hours on two consecutive nights, and then their hormone levels and hunger ratings were recorded. Findings showed that the hormone leptin, which alerts the brain that it is time to stop eating, was 18 percent lower than before the experiment, whereas the hormone ghrelin, which triggers hunger, was 28 percent higher. The men also showed a 24-percent increase in their self-assessed "hunger rating" following the sleep restriction.[2]

- The rise in obesity has occurred simultaneously with the decline in time spent sleeping, with only about 25 percent of young Americans currently getting eight to nine hours of sleep per night, as compared to 41 percent in 1960.[3]

- Inadequate sleep can have disastrous effects on your weight-loss efforts, impair your concentration, and even mimic the symptoms of impaired glucose tolerance (which can lead to diabetes and hypertension).

- Your mood suffers when you don't get enough shut-eye, causing you to become disoriented on the job, fatigued behind the wheel, or irritated at home. These mood swings can affect your relationships with others and even lead to depression.

To help you sleep, try creating a sleep-friendly environment by using your bedroom only as a sleep sanctuary. Avoid using your bedroom to pay bills, do homework, watch television, eat, or talk on the phone. Equip your room with soft lighting, comfortable bedding, and relaxing music. Lower the temperature a few notches, and turn the clock away from your view.

Remember that sleep is a time of rest and healing that prepares you for the next day's challenges and brings mental focus and consistency to your program and goals. The more your body gets into the rhythm of regular sleep, the more the rest of your life can find a similar, consistent rhythm. In fact, consistently getting at least eight hours of sleep may be one of the easiest lifestyle changes you can make to help you maintain a healthy weight.

Action Step: For the next two weeks, try to do just that—get seven to eight hours of sleep per night.

WEEK 2 REVIEW

As your coach, we've introduced you to a lot of new material to help you fuel your great adventure. You may not have realized it yet, but you're already well on your way. Feel the new spring in your step, the lift in your mood, the sense that you count on yourself as you head toward a destination full of promise and reward.

In the next week we will introduce action steps that will make it even easier for you to stick to your goals in the upcoming weeks and years!

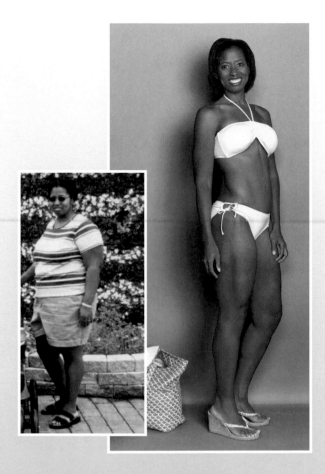

BIRDIE VARNEDORE
Miami, Florida
35 years old
Highest Weight: 292 pounds
Weight Lost: 143 pounds
http://my.sparkpeople.com/MOM5INFL

"I can't pinpoint one particular reason for losing weight. As a physician, I knew my weight was unhealthy and it would eventually lead to medical problems. To be there for my five children, I knew I had to get healthy. I was embarrassed by my size. I felt that being obese showed that my life was out of control.

"I have referred SparkPeople to hundreds of patients. I remember how painful it was to be obese, so I can't sit by and let them suffer when there's hope."

Birdie is the ultimate motivator. She appeared in People *magazine in a feature celebrating her success. She was also able to share her inspiring story and tips with millions of viewers on* Good Morning America.

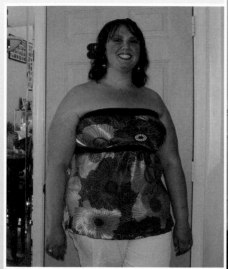
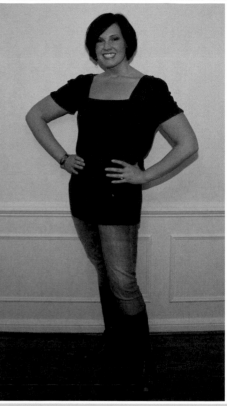

BRANDY BLACKBURN
Charlottesville, Virginia
24 years old
Highest Weight: 335 pounds
Weight Lost: 172 pounds
http://my.sparkpeople.com/BBANGEL1214

"I broke down in an amusement park (after not fitting in a ride) and started thinking about all I had missed out on because of my weight. I didn't want my daughter to be ashamed of me, and I didn't want her to go through what I did. I decided that day to make a change—to be a good example for not only my daughter but also all the kids I teach.

"I began going to the gym three times a week for 30 minutes. I couldn't run at all, and riding the bike for 20 minutes exhausted me. Now I work out five days a week for an hour. I was never able to run a mile, so to be training for 5Ks is shocking. It's funny that something I dreaded so much is now a passion of mine."

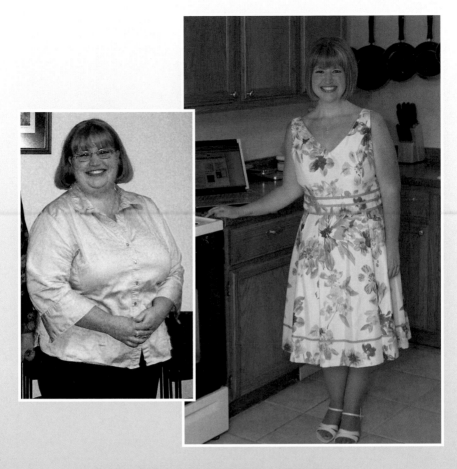

CHASITY SCHOONOVER
Wichita, Kansas
33 years old
Highest Weight: 250 pounds
Weight Lost: 111 pounds
http://my.sparkpeople.com/CHASITY_ANN

"My brother joined SparkPeople to lose weight, and I decided that if he could do it, I could, too! During the time I was losing weight, I lost two grandparents, which was a huge challenge. I am a comfort eater and also a perfectionist. To recognize that I would have bad days was hard, but I learned to forgive myself and get back to work. That was a *huge* step. I couldn't have made this journey without my faith, family, and friends!

"Since losing weight, I'm happier and more energetic, optimistic, outgoing, and confident. I sleep better, feel better, and can walk across the room without being winded. For the first time, I actually have a life—and I love living it."

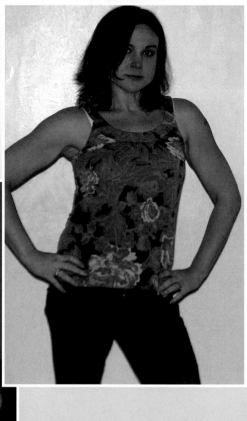

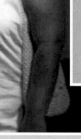

DANA CHRISTINE
Dagsboro, Delaware
28 years old
Highest Weight: 300 pounds
Weight Lost: 154 pounds
http://my.sparkpeople.com/DANACHRISTINE

"I've been heavy my entire life. I weighed 230 pounds by the time I was 12. I felt hopeless, not knowing where to go or what to do, and this feeling persisted for years. In 2008, I had a miscarriage, and when I looked at the doctor's chart it said that I was 'morbidly obese.' I couldn't believe it. I was 300 pounds, and I knew I was heavy, but *morbidly obese!?!* This was the turning point in my life.

"If I can lose the weight, anyone can. I was addicted to fast food and anything chocolate before I discovered SparkPeople. I started in April 2008, and I have been on the Website every day since! I used to look through the motivation stories of others and dream of being one of them. And now I am!"

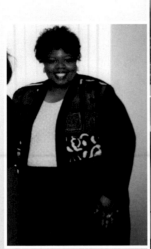

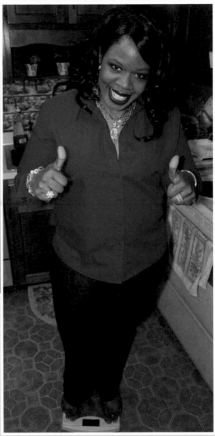

DEONDRA WARDELLE
Louisville, Kentucky
38 years old
Highest Weight: 407 pounds
Weight Lost: 170 pounds
http://my.sparkpeople.com/D710DANCE

"I was miserable. My joints ached, and it was hard to catch my breath after walking even short distances. My biggest challenge is to not be discouraged by setbacks. You must be patient and resolve that, no matter what, you will make this lifestyle change work—one decision at a time. My biggest motivators are my faith and the pages and blogs of other SparkPeople.

"When I hit 407 pounds, I knew it was only a matter of time before my habits affected my health even more drastically. Since starting SparkPeople, my life has changed dramatically. Now I am more active and have more energy. And I'm on a mission to motivate anyone I come in contact with."

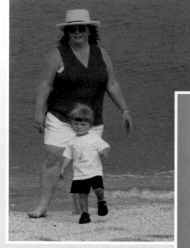

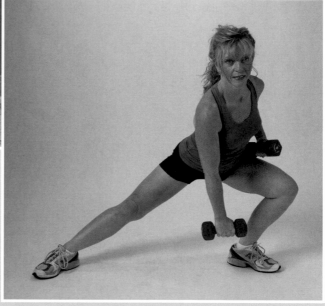

ELLENMARY DETORE
Freehold, New Jersey
43 years old
Highest Weight: 230 pounds
Weight Lost: 105 pounds
http://my.sparkpeople.com/SAMSON94

"I was diagnosed with lupus in 1992 and put on medication that slowed my metabolism. I found SparkPeople totally by accident, and I was blown away. All of this information and people just like me were together in one place. This really helped me take control and learn the right way to do things.

"The challenge of battling both my weight and my disease makes me even more proud of my accomplishments. And my doctor told me that my new lifestyle helped put the lupus in remission! My life has changed dramatically. I am more confident, and I like to challenge myself to accomplish new goals. For example, I started singing and am now in the process of making a demo."

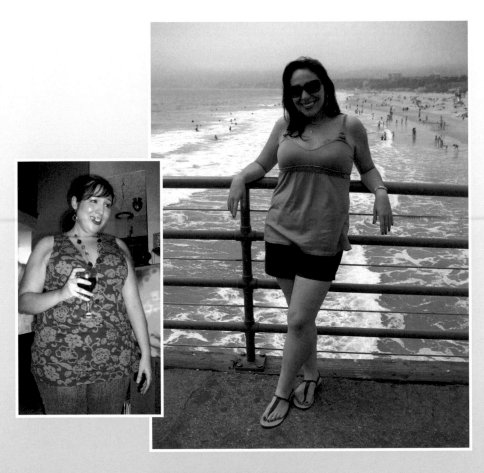

ERIN MUSQUIZ

Dallas, Texas
27 years old
Highest Weight: 201 pounds
Weight Lost: 37 pounds
http://my.sparkpeople.com/ERINALEXIS20

"Life for me before weight loss was tiring and frustrating. My hips hurt when I sat, my feet and knees hurt when I walked, I felt un-girly, and life simply wasn't fun. The saddest part of it all is that I felt much older than my 27 years.

"I love SparkPeople so much that I've inspired my best friend to lose 50 pounds, my mom to lose 13, my aunt to lose 15, and my boyfriend to lose 25! I couldn't have done any of that without SparkPeople. I look forward to spinning the wheel, watching my SparkPoints go up, up, up and my weight go down, down, down!"

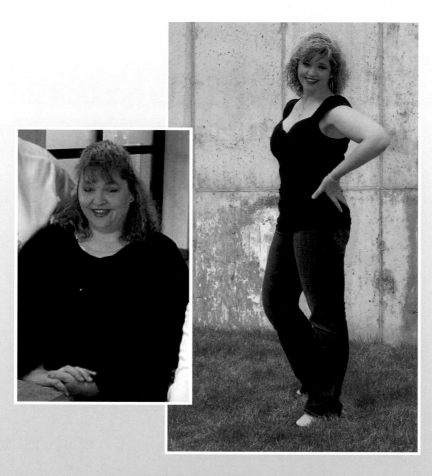

FLOSSIE ALEXANDER
Wichita, Kansas
37 years old
Highest Weight: 325 pounds
Weight Lost: 165 pounds
http://my.sparkpeople.com/FLORENCEOSI

"I tried one fad diet after another, and in 2006, I reached the end of my rope. I joined a medically supervised weight-loss clinic, spending nearly $800 a month. With seven kids, I couldn't continue with the clinic. With our food bill going up and the economy going down, we were feeling the squeeze.

"In January 2008, a friend introduced me to SparkPeople. After joining, I found invaluable tools to help with my weight-loss journey. Healthy recipes for the whole family cut down on our overall food bill because I could plan the week ahead and shop for deals. My kids have become educated right along with me, and their choices in life will be better than mine."

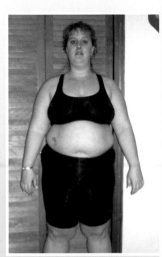
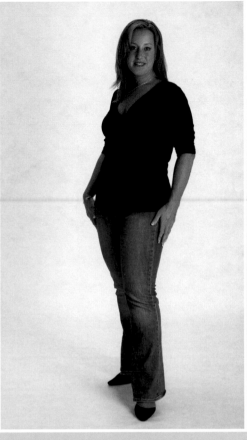

HEATHER HOLLOWAY
Hartford, Connecticut
36 years old
Highest Weight: 240 pounds
Weight Lost: 104 pounds
http://my.sparkpeople.com/PUMPKINFACE73

"My turning point was when I realized I couldn't walk up a flight of stairs without being winded. I knew then that I had to take control of my health. My biggest inspiration is my daughter, because I want to be the best mom and role model I can be. I ran my first race with my daughter by my side. She gave me the courage to push myself and helped me believe in myself.

"My next goal is to complete a triathlon. I have always loved to swim. In 2008, I took up biking in August and running in September. Never in my wildest dreams did I think I would be standing here today ready and able to compete in such an event."

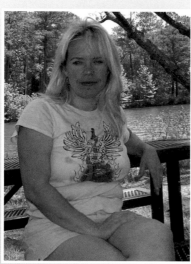
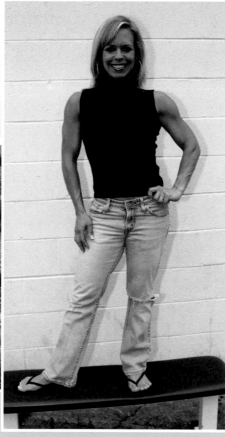

KIM MITCHELL
Virginia Beach, Virginia
38 years old
Highest Weight: 158 pounds
Weight Lost: 29 pounds
http://my.sparkpeople.com/URBANMOMMY

"Over the past 20 years, I tried many different weight-loss plans. Every kind of diet, every kind of exercise—but the truth is, I was never serious enough to make a change. However, I was desperate to try whatever was out there.

"After losing weight, I became much more confident and excited about pursuing a fitness lifestyle. I have become a certified personal trainer, a bodybuilder, and President of TransFigure Fitness, LLC. Now I teach others how to plan out healthy meals and train with purpose and intensity so they can achieve similar success. And I demonstrate, in NPC physique competitions, how commitment and consistency do pay off."

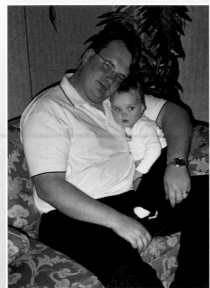
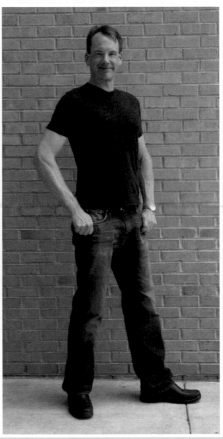

GREGORY GAUL
Topeka, Kansas
35 years old
Highest Weight: 350 pounds
Weight Lost: 135 pounds
http://my.sparkpeople.com/KSIGMA1222

"The funeral of my best friend's dad forced me to go back to my hometown and see people I hadn't seen for 15 years. His family spoke of how he always saw the potential in people and always wanted to bring that out in others. I left feeling deeply inspired. I focused my pain and mourning into inspiration and told myself I was going to change.

"I started by eating three healthy meals a day. This was something I hadn't done since I was a teenager. I rarely ate breakfast or lunch, and I had a large dinner after work. I would be so hungry that all I did until I went to bed was eat. I am much more active, and I find that I have a better outlook on everything. I love my life now."

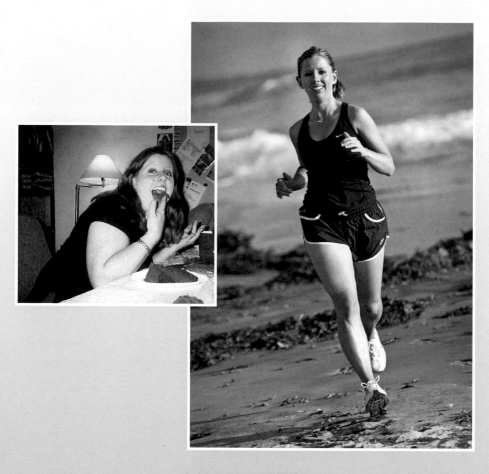

LEAH REED
San Diego, California
30 years old
Highest Weight: 186 pounds
Weight Lost: 62 pounds
http://my.sparkpeople.com/SPRING4FAL

"There was an incident on the freeway where a woman got upset with me, so she made a pig face at me. It was a blunt statement that I was fat. I hated the fact that she was right, and I wanted to take back the power I had given away by allowing my weight to get out of control.

"Wrapping my head around the fact that, in order to be successful in the long run, this had to be a lifestyle change was a major challenge for me. Now I can't imagine living any other way. I started running about seven months ago and have since run my first half marathon and full marathon! I look forward to seeing what the future has in store for me! Nothing can stop me now!"

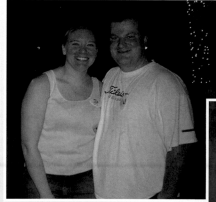

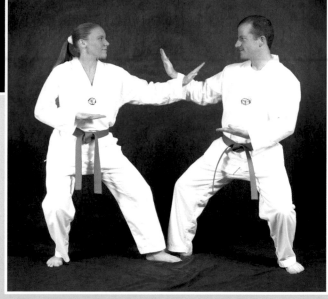

MATT AND DENISE TAUSIG
Lake Ozark, Missouri
32, and 30 years old
Highest Weights: 265 and 175 pounds
Weight Lost: 80 and 35 pounds
http://my.sparkpeople.com/GOLFPRO
http://my.sparkpeople.com/DENISE_SP

"Our lives used to revolve around eating out. Unfortunately this kind of lifestyle left us weighing more than ever. We enjoyed life, but we definitely weren't happy with our appearances. Both our families have a history of poor health and obesity. It was time for a change.

"Learning to live more healthfully changed our lives. We enrolled in martial arts, which boosted our confidence and discipline. We also started eating at home more often and making healthier food choices. Beyond the nutrition and fitness advice, SparkPeople helped us understand how setting goals can help us achieve anything we want."

Matt and Denise were so active helping people in the SparkPeople community that Denise is now an employee of the company!

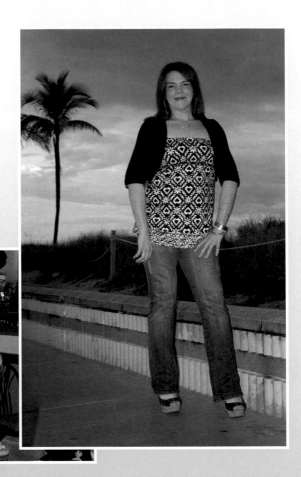

MELISSA PEREZ-LETTS
Fort Lauderdale, Florida
26 years old
Highest Weight: 330 pounds
Weight Lost: 186 pounds
http://my.sparkpeople.com/URBANNENA

"I was e-mailing pictures to my grandfather, and I came across a recent photo of myself. I was so big I didn't even recognize myself. At that very moment, I got up, with my regular clothes on, and started exercising.

"SparkPeople has been a lifesaver. What helped me out at first was setting mini-goals, simple things like listening to a motivating song or drinking more water. Having someone there to share common goals or mishaps was incredibly helpful. The motivation and inspiration I got was overwhelming. My life has changed completely. I am now a personal trainer, and I am studying to be an R.N., with the ultimate goal of becoming a nurse anesthetist."

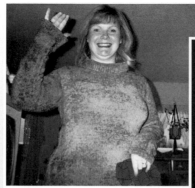

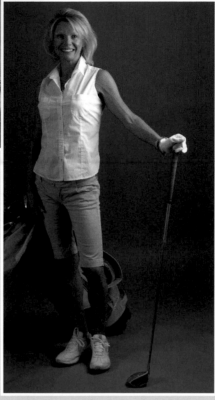

VICKI LYNN
Sault Sainte Marie, Canada
38 years old
Highest Weight: 229 pounds
Weight Lost: 108 pounds
http://my.sparkpeople.com/PINKJEWEL2002

"I had tried quite a few diets, but I couldn't stick to one for long. I even tried Wii Fit. When I stood on the board to set up my character, I watched in horror as she ballooned up in size and the cute little voice said, 'That's obese.' I stared at the weight display and had a breakdown. I had to change.

"Since losing weight, I'm not as self-conscious, and I've noticed I'm kinder to others. I have a passion for fun fitness and delicious healthy eating. And now I can give my boys childhood memories that focus on fun times we spend camping, biking, walking, and talking. I will teach them to make healthy choices so they won't have to endure the issues I did."

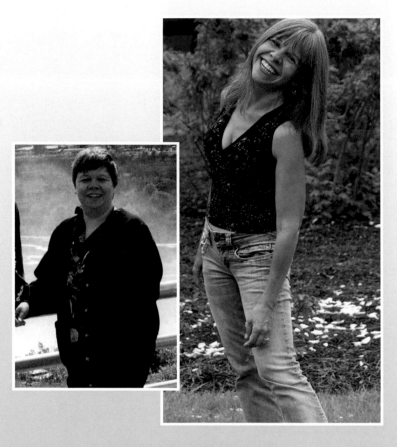

VIVIAN BEDOYA
New Brunswick, New Jersey
50 years old
Highest Weight: 153 pounds
Weight Lost: 54 pounds
http://my.sparkpeople.com/BEMORESTUBBORN

"At about five feet, I was fairly rotund at my highest weight. However, once I began making progress, I was pleased to discover that my health issues were completely gone or alleviated. As a bonus, I discovered that I love running—something I *never* dreamed I would enjoy.

"As glad as I am about my success, it is the success of my daughters that makes me happiest. My daughters, Jessica and Lisette, have lost 45 and 80 pounds respectively and made health a priority. That I motivated them through my example is wonderful; that they took that example and through their actions and commitment created their own success is a priceless legacy!"

CHAPTER 8

STAGE 3: LIFESTYLE CHANGE

When an athlete first starts out, she needs a coach to manage and motivate her, provide her with knowledge and basic skills, and offer her guidance in facing setbacks. But as the athlete gains more experience, she learns to incorporate the coach's techniques into her own personal arsenal. Eventually she no longer needs a full-time coach to wake her up for a game, to stand over her while she does push-ups, or to call out inspiration. She's learned how to do it for herself.

In Week 2, we acted as your coach, but now we're going to pass the baton and teach you how to become one for yourself. Just think about what a great coach can do for an athlete or a team. The coach can figure out the right buttons to push to help the person or team reach accomplishments they might not have thought possible. We want to help you learn the strategies and techniques that a great coach uses to do this so you can motivate yourself. But don't worry—we're not going to leave you alone. We'll still be right there behind you, offering support and advice and a safety net in case you fall.

Many diets are fleeting relationships. There's no coach at all, just a set of rules telling you what you should and shouldn't eat. As far as diets are concerned, it's all about the scale. Follow these rules until the numbers drop, then you're on your own. It's at this crucial juncture that most people revert to the habits that were causing them to gain weight in the first place and enter the yo-yo diet cycle.

Not this time.

We promise that you can set yourself free from "dieting" and change your life, just like our member WAVES did:

> *I have always struggled with my weight. My self-confidence was extremely low. After having my two children I gained so much weight I*

thought it would never come off. I tried everything. Now, I have lost 50 pounds! I feel great and have never gotten so many compliments in my lifetime. I feel like a changed person with a new outlook on life. I don't see this as a diet anymore. To me the word diet means "struggle." This is a way of life for me now. THANK YOU!

Our major goal this week is to dramatically increase your odds of incorporating the SparkPeople program as a permanent healthy lifestyle change. Regularly using these techniques we'll show you in this chapter can change the course of your life.

WEEK 3 ACTION STEPS

This week we want you to continue performing and tracking each of the action steps from Week 2. These will become easier and easier as you adjust to this new way of living. This week's action steps are specifically designed to give you even more motivation to keep reaching your goals. Integrating the healthy habits with the motivational techniques that make them stick is a powerful combination that can make a major difference in your life.

This week, you'll do the following action steps:

1. Continue with SparkTime
2. Review your goals
3. Choose at least one motivational technique and incorporate it into your week
4. Choose at least one way to draw support from positive people
5. Learn how to overcome hurdles

TAKE SPARKTIME

In the Fast Break, we introduced the idea of SparkTime—a period you take each day to think about your goals and how you plan to schedule them into your life. We love the idea of reserving some special time each day just for you.

We know that our online members often log in every day to give themselves this crucial focus. Offline, you might sit down with your calendar and your morning coffee (or better yet, your morning cup of water!), or take a moment before bedtime with your tracker or journal, to focus on how things went that day and to plan for the day ahead.

During my SparkTime in the morning, I like to review my goals and also plan out my day. I have a checklist of regular items I do each day—from a reminder to plan my daily workout to some of the motivational techniques listed below. This checklist helps me prepare to make each day a great one!

Action Step: Make time each day to sit down and review your progress, focus on your goals, and think about the positive things that have happened in your life.

REVIEW YOUR GOALS FOR MOTIVATION

People often set goals, then release them like helium balloons when they become overwhelmed with other pressing activities. Before they know it, the goals have floated off, indistinct and far away. At SparkPeople, we know that keeping your goals in front of you is key. Simply looking at your goals serves as a powerful motivator.

I often say that once people truly know the real reason why they want to make a healthy lifestyle change—the ultimate goal is almost never just "to lose 30 pounds"—then they are so much more likely to make the healthy lifestyle change *and* reach their most important goals. Talk about a "win/win"!

In the Fast Break, you completed your vision collage and placed goal reminders in key places. Now make certain that you're looking at these regularly throughout the day. These collages and goals reminders should be so thoroughly integrated into your life that they provide you with effortless and continuous motivation.

Action Step: Look at your goals every day. Visualize reaching those goals and how you will feel. This should take no more than a few minutes each day.

GET MOTIVATED

Our motivational strategies are easy and fun to follow. They provide fuel to your program and act as glue to make your healthy habits stick.

This week we want you to adopt one or more of the following techniques:

1. Positive self-talk
2. Motivational moments
3. Journal writing
4. Streaks
5. Rewards

We've developed many options to choose from because we know that different people are motivated in different ways. And different techniques work better at certain

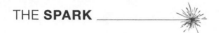

times in your life. Read on to learn more about each of these options. Over time, you can try them all to find which works best for you.

Action Step: Choose at least one motivation technique and use it this week to help you stay on track.

Give Yourself a Pep Talk

When I face a challenge, I'll often take just a few moments to give myself a pep talk. When I do this, I draw on the power of all the goals I've reached in the past to tell myself that I know I can meet this challenge. This is a great way to be not only my own coach, but also my own cheerleader.

In fact, the number-one motivational strategy of successful members in our Secrets of Success survey was "I give myself positive self-talk." Studies show that positive self-talk is extremely effective in changing our attitudes and mood. Our polls bear this out: quite simply, you can change who you are by changing what you say to yourself.

It's easy to be self-critical, to barrage yourself with negative self-talk, compare yourself with everyone else, mentally beat yourself up, or put yourself down. But these negative thoughts and feelings mean that you're working against, not for, yourself.

Break this cycle by turning your goals into positive affirmations or mantras that you say aloud to help take control of your thoughts and attitudes. When they are repeated daily, they tend to reprogram your thinking.

Be aware of the self-fulfilling words and thoughts that can wander around your mind: *I never succeed. I have no willpower. I'm never a success at anything.* How do these words make you feel? Pretty rotten and discouraged. Intervene on your own behalf to halt these self-wounding messages. Try replacing negative thoughts with positive affirmations, such as: *I'm strong and motivated. I'm making progress. I had trouble today, but I'll improve tomorrow.*

Other members, like JIMSRAINBOW, have come to rely on pep talk to meet their goals and get through difficult times, not just with their weight loss but in life.

> *Sometimes, the only way I can get through a night is by telling myself about the accomplishments, however few or small, that I've had. It works like magic. But I thought I was going a little nuts, talking to myself on the treadmill, telling myself it's the last mile, verbally patting myself on the back whenever I started to feel low. Thank you for showing me that I'm actually on the right track with all the self pep talk.*

SOME SPARKPEOPLE MEMBER MANTRAS

You don't drown by falling in the water, only by staying there. — NEWME086

For the victim, only excuses. For the warrior, no excuses! — BETHK

Something the coach said in John Irving's The Hotel New Hampshire. *"You've got to get obsessed and stay obsessed."* — SPARKLESSENCE

Since I've been running lately, when I feel like I want to give up and slow down the pace, I just keep thinking, "I will not give up on myself." — LUVME

I CAN, I AM, I WILL, and IF not today . . . when? — THEMOTIVATOR1

Today is my new beginning (I say this every day). — 4NUMBERS

A bikini! A bikini before I die! — WORKINGFORME

Embrace Motivational Moments

Other people's lives matter to us; we're inspired by their examples of courage and perseverance. Exposing yourself to motivational and inspirational stories—whether they're directly related to weight loss and getting fit or about accomplishing other great goals—is a powerful tool.

In our Secrets of Success survey, the most successful members reported using the inspirational strategies that we call "motivational moments." For example, of 100-pound losers, 71 percent read inspiring stories on SparkPeople.com, and over 60 percent regularly read motivational stories and books and watched motivational movies and films to keep themselves inspired.

In our survey, even we were a little surprised at how much people utilized these tools and how highly they correlate with success. The key is converting the power of these motivational moments to help power your overall program.

How many times have you watched an inspirational movie or heard a rousing speaker and felt as if you were ready to move mountains? But then a few hours or days later you were back into your normal routine with no lasting changes. Now we want you to be more mindful and cherishing of these moments. Notice whenever you're moved by a speech, a book, a movie, or a special experience. Write about it in your journal so you can hold on to the power of your inspired feelings.

Read about Other People's Success

Reading about the bravery and perseverance of my own personal heroes—from Viktor Frankl to Ernest Shackleton—has had a huge impact on my own life. So it was no surprise to me that the number-one technique our 100-pound losers used was reading other people's inspiring stories of successful weight loss and of reaching health, fitness, and other life goals. You, too, can benefit from these success stories by logging on to our online book program at SparkPeople.com/TheSpark.

Watch an Inspiring Movie

Who said changing your lifestyle is all work and no play? The best part of drawing inspiration from a movie is that there's one out there for everyone. Some of us draw inspiration from cheering for the underdogs, especially in sports films. Others find inspiration in stories of courage or of triumphing over personal setbacks. A movie conjures emotions unlike any other form of entertainment, making us understand what the characters are going through and how we can aspire to be more like them. You'll find a few suggestions in the box to the right, but feel free to pick your own.

MOTIVATING MOVIES

Stand and Deliver
The Shawshank Redemption
Mr. Holland's Opus
Apollo 13
Simon Birch
Patch Adams
Rudy
October Sky
Rocky
Big Fish
The Bucket List
The Pianist
It's a Wonderful Life

Be Inspired by Music

Staying motivated by music is one of the most common inspirational techniques successful SparkPeople use. Music is such a powerful motivator because it can reach out and touch your soul and move you to take action—all with only a few minutes of beautiful, melodic sound.

Build a list of motivational songs. Listen to one of your favorites as you get up in the morning and let it "ring" in your head throughout the day. It can be as energizing as a morning cup of coffee. Music is also a great way to prevent boredom. Download a few new songs to jazz up your next trip on the treadmill!

Read an Inspiring Quote

When you need a jolt of inspiration, take note of the wisdom of others. Meaningful quotations may only take a few seconds to read, but they can have lasting effects on your mood and performance. Go to the bookstore or library and leaf through books of quotations or check out SparkPeople's motivational quotes, along with commentary, online at SparkPeople.com/resource/quotes.asp. Once you find a quote that works for you, use it. Hang it on your mirror. Keep a copy in your wallet. Tape it to your computer monitor.

QUOTES TO LIVE BY

Remember to live.
Better to light a candle than to curse the darkness.
Never confuse a single defeat with a final defeat.
Stand for something or fall for anything.
Who I am really keeps surprising me.
From a tiny spark may burst a mighty flame.

Write in a Journal

Writing in a journal is a great way to learn more about yourself. Here are two types of journal entries to consider:

- *Action journal.* An inspiring way to keep track of your weight-loss experience is to keep a before-during-and-after journal that chronicles your journey to a new, healthy lifestyle. If you're already keeping a journal or using one to track your food intake, you can use the same book to record your whole experience this way. Include writing and photos from all stages, showing how you felt and looked all along the way. This can end up being a mini-autobiography, a book of your life that traces your challenges and commemorates your success.

- *Success journal.* Another idea is to keep a journal that focuses on all the positives in your life—a place where you record what you're proud of and what you've accomplished. Think back as far as you can, and record often. One technique is to write down a highlight from every day. The more you focus on what you are good at, what you have done, and what you are capable of, the more motivated you'll be.

Streak for Motivation

Remember streaks? They are the sustained, consistent, positive activities that are one of the most crucial elements of our program.

Streaks are motivational powerhouses: small daily and weekly goals that help launch your program and keep it alive. Continuing a streak—whether it's tracking your food every day, doing ten minutes of daily exercise, or drinking an extra cup of water—gives you the kind of satisfaction and motivation that will build confidence and momentum and fuel your journey.

How to Do a Streak

Set a definite time period for your streak, such as "I'm going to cut out soda for a month," instead of leaving it open-ended. If you reach that goal and want to continue the streak, just keep it going with a new goal, or move on to a streak on a different topic if you'd like.

Start with something you feel sure you can succeed with but don't already do regularly. If the idea of doing something every day is intimidating and stressful, try a weekly streak, such as "I'll walk three times a week every week for two months." Keep track of the number of weeks in a row you reach this goal. A variation is to give yourself one or two free passes each week, so that missing a day or two doesn't derail you. Reward yourself along the way as you reach streak milestones, especially when you reach your streak goal (a month without soda) or a personal best (the longest you've ever gone without soda). Creating positive peer pressure by streaking in public! Telling others of your streak will help you follow through, plus it gives them the opportunity to help.

If you miss a day and break your streak, don't worry. Just reset your counter and try to outdo yourself next time. Streaks aren't about perfection. The important thing with streaks is to figure out how to make them work for you. Some people love this strategy and will do just about anything to keep their streaks alive; others don't like the pressure.

While it's common to reward yourself when you reach a goal weight or accomplish a fitness feat, sometimes it's even more motivating to reward yourself for the journey, not just the destination. Seeing how consistently you've been taking steps to reach a goal (and knowing others can see it, too) can help boost your resolve and keep your motivation going strong. This is especially true when you've done your part but the scale hasn't budged, even though you've been making the right choices every day. That's why we created SparkStreaks—an online SparkPeople tracking tool that can motivate you to stay on track and help you reach some amazing goals! You can find a link to SparkStreaks from the online book program at SparkPeople.com/TheSpark.

Using our online tracker, you'll be able to see your own progress, which will help increase your accountability and help you stick to your goals.

Reward Yourself

Everyone deserves a pat on the back once in a while. And there's no better time to get one than when you're out of your comfort zone, challenging yourself to improve. Our most successful members think and act in positive ways, patting themselves on the back and applauding their own efforts. Over half of those who lost 100 pounds or more (54 percent) reward themselves when they reach a goal or adopt a healthy habit.

SPARKPEOPLE REWARDS ROSTER

Here are a few of the rewards that SparkPeople members have developed. You can choose any or all of these reward ideas as you move through the program—or add your own—and use them liberally. Be creative. Make it fun!

- Compliment yourself. Write down what you would say to anyone else who accomplished what you have.

- Arrange a buddy reward system with a friend—offer to babysit, walk a dog, or wash a car for each other when one of you reaches a goal.

- Put $1 in a jar every time you meet a goal. When it reaches $50, treat yourself.

- Create a "trophy scrapbook" where you keep mementos from your accomplishments.

- Make a grab bag of little prizes. When you reach a significant goal, reach in and get your reward!

- Subscribe to a magazine you've always wanted.

- Go canoeing or do something outdoors.

- Celebrate "100 Percent Days." If you reach 100 percent of your goals that day, choose two rewards.

- Carve out some time to be by yourself.

- Enjoy the special event you've been working toward—like your daughter's wedding or a school reunion.

- Take a vacation or weekend getaway. Vacations are the crown jewels of rewards, creating anticipation and memories that can last for months.

Setting up your own personal rewards system is another great way of becoming your own best coach. Now you'll always have something to shoot for as you continue on your journey. It's like playing a game where you collect different "goodies" along the way.

You can reward yourself for anything you please. The keys to doing it right are consistency and frequency. Remember, you're building a lifestyle full of healthy habits, and habits require repetition. That means rewarding good actions when they occur, instead of saving all of your rewards until you reach your goal results. The best approach is a mix: Use rewards tied to longer-range weight milestones to maintain some big-picture motivation. At the same time, use rewards tied to daily and weekly actions to give those healthy habits some positive reinforcement along the way.

Large rewards such as vacations or new clothes work great as "goal rewards," what you give yourself for reaching your major weight goal. Small rewards are perfect as regular, everyday "action rewards." These are the rewards you give yourself every day for meeting your calorie levels, walking or running an extra half-mile, consistently eating your veggies, or simply following your meal plan. Remember, it's every bit as crucial to reward behaviors and habits as it is to reward results. Small rewards can range from watching a movie or giving yourself a compliment to pausing for 20 minutes to call a friend or take a bubble bath.

Above all, make the reward personally meaningful. A new pair of shoes may not hold as much motivation as a night alone with a book. Also, be honest with yourself. Fudging the numbers mentally or "borrowing" against the next reward hurts the cause of building a lifetime habit. Remember to keep your focus on building a habit, not just figuring out how to get the reward.

An object may have more meaning if you give it to yourself as a reward. For example, if you buy yourself new piece of jewelry when you reach a meaningful goal, then anytime you wear that jewelry you'll be reminded of the goal you met. This is a fun way to surround yourself with motivation!

This strategy works even better when you make it official. Write down your rewards. Record what behavior or goal you're working toward (and when you want to reach it, if it is a goal that can be scheduled), then tell others! Also, plan to celebrate, either by yourself or with others.

Here are some great ways that some of our members have rewarded themselves:

> *I'm pretty sentimental, and I love it when my seven-year-old makes stuff for me. I think he'd be excited to be part of this and make me a "trophy" (i.e., a picture) every time I get to another milestone. Then I could hang them on the wall together. He loves to come to my office and hang pictures. I could have a trophy wall, or something, and every time I reward myself for something, I could have him make me a trophy to add to my trophy wall . . . then I'm involving my family in my goals. — ZOOFAN*

I have a grab bag of sorts. I gave all my friends $5, and they could buy me anything they wanted . . . They wrap it and put it in a box that I keep at work so I'm not tempted to peek—and the people with whom I work contributed to it also. When I reach the next ten pounds lost, I get to reach in and pull out a surprise! It keeps me motivated to continue with my new lifestyle. — MAURIZIA

I am on a tight budget and never "waste" money on myself. I buy the best oil, gas, etc. for my car, the best for my family . . . but I just started understanding how important I am and am starting to treat myself well. I bought myself trail shoes to hike and will be buying some new shorts too. Buying workout clothes with good breathing material rather than my dorky shorts is my new way to show myself that I do deserve to be rewarded for all the positive changes I have made. Good job, self! — BRICKYJR

As a therapist and a psych instructor, I know rewards/positive reinforcement work much better than punishment and the changes are longer lasting, but I didn't always practice what I preach! Take heart, members, this does work better, research backs it up! — JAXMOMMY

Online Rewards

If you choose to use the SparkPeople Website, you'll see that we have built rewards into the site, including virtual trophies for reaching different SparkPoints levels and graphics to display when you've lost weight at different milestones (5, 10, 20, 50 pounds). You can also save up your SparkPoints to "buy" virtual gifts to reward yourself and congratulate other members.

THE POWER OF POSITIVE PEOPLE

At SparkPeople, we celebrate a fundamental truth—that humans need each other, perhaps never so much as when we're trying to change our lives. The hallmark of our program is community. We believe in the power of connection to sustain us, uplift us, and help us thrive. In this week, we focus on how you can ask for and receive support from others. In the next week, we'll turn it around and discuss how you can spread the spark to others.

A recent study published by the *New England Journal of Medicine* showed that a person's chance of becoming obese increased by 57 percent if he or she had a friend who became obese during a given time period.[1] If the friend was of the same sex, the odds of becoming obese jumped by 71 percent. But the second part of the study was even more fascinating to us at SparkPeople. It turned out that if, on the other hand, a person associated with others committed to losing weight, the odds of slimming down likewise increased significantly.

Of course, we didn't need a study to prove that healthy and fit friends can make you healthy and fit too. We witness this all the time, firsthand. Such friends can act as powerful motivators, not only by their own great example, but by providing a helping hand, an experienced ear, and inspiring words to fire you up, pick you back up, and help keep you going.

Tap into the Power!

You may not think of people as nourishing, but indeed they are. Just notice how different you feel after getting together with an optimistic, encouraging friend, as opposed to a negative, self-involved one. Our SparkPeople members realize this and regularly tap into the power of positive people as a potent motivational tool. Sixty percent of successful members connect with positive people who they know will help them stay positive, and 58.6 percent proactively read other people's success stories to stay motivated. Of 100-pound losers, the numbers are even higher—72 percent of those people proactively connect with positive people who they know will keep them positive, and 71 percent read inspiring stories of other successful SparkPeople.

We know about the power of positive self-talk, but what better way to reinforce it than by adding a choir of encouragement from others?

Your Friends Can Make You Thin and Healthy

Surround yourself with positive and healthy influences. Nearly 60 percent of SparkPeople members who lost at least 100 pounds had six or more healthy friends—those who supported their healthy lifestyle through encouragement or active participation. Healthy friends provide the motivation to continue when you are down and companionship in a struggle where you could feel alone.

In addition to the number of healthy friends you have, it also matters how often you're in touch with them. Most successful members—over 65 percent of them—were engaged with their healthy friends daily, while another 27 percent were engaged weekly or several times a week. They kept in touch in a variety of ways—in person (82 percent), by e-mail (70 percent), by phone (57 percent) and in online forums (57 percent). The majority also belonged to at least one SparkTeam. And more than 50 percent belonged to five or more SparkTeams!

It's Okay to Ask for Help

People often treat their weight-loss issues as an affliction that should be hidden, and their weight loss efforts as a private, embarrassing endeavor. But if you're serious about attaining long-term results, it's time to come out of quarantine and let someone in on the secret.

You may feel shy asking for help, but you'll be surprised by how eager most people are to join in and lend a hand—or even jump on the healthy-living bandwagon themselves. Working with others can also accelerate your progress and make your journey more pleasurable. Having someone by your side, facing challenges with you, can help you strive, survive, and celebrate. Is there a more rewarding way to lose weight?

Besides, involving others is proven to work. A University of Pittsburgh study showed that dieters who had just one other person check in on their progress lost twice as much weight as those who didn't have help.[2] As the researchers said, "social support adds accountability."

Get Others Involved

Even the greatest athletes in the world can't do it alone. That's why they surround themselves with coaches, mentors, trainers, teammates, partners, and fans.

Your weight-loss goals are every bit as important as those of a world-class athlete. This is why SparkPeople emphasizes meeting and getting to know other members, or reaching out and connecting with friends, neighbors, family, or others in your own communities.

People naturally perform better when others are on their side. Even in everyday nutrition and fitness, we've found that people who involve others and ask for help achieve much better results and stick to their programs longer than people who try to go the distance on their own.

Why is that? For starters, positive peer pressure can be one of the most powerful motivators around. It's tougher to quit when someone else is counting on you. In fact, with a team that's pulling for you, it's less likely that you'll *want* to quit.

When you involve others, you have access to more knowledge, ideas, enthusiasm, and resources. And having other people help out just makes weight loss a lot more fun.

Here are some possible ways to get people to help without making large demands on their time:

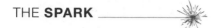

- Ask a friend to check with you once a week to see how you're doing.

- Ask your significant other to be there when you need to unload.

- Ask a co-worker to keep you upbeat.

- Ask your kids to help you find active ways to have fun.

- Ask your mom to pass along inspirational reading and interesting health news.

- Ask a friend to take "before" and "in-progress" photos.

- Ask a friend to be your fitness buddy—someone with whom you can agree to helping each other reach consistent goals with friendly encouragement and regular contact.

KRISTYMOM located that special someone to help cheer her on—right in her own house:

I found one person in my life, my 15-year-old daughter, Kristy. She has been my inspiration. She has stuck with me through everything—every tear—every craving—walking with me, tennis lessons, running. She holds my hand when I get upset, cheers me on, encourages me. Loves me. Without her, I probably would have given up a couple of times. I have lost 60 percent of my original body weight, and will not go back. She has shown me I can do anything. Find that one person, even in a group of 100 doubters.

Online Community

Sometimes it's even easier to find support online. While you won't have the benefit of someone meeting you at the corner for a morning walk, you will have access to practically unlimited numbers of people who share your goals and are often available online 24/7.

The SparkPeople.com online community is a perfect example of what can happen when a large group of people band together and build a healthy environment. When you're posting on the support message boards, you're never alone. Someone is always there to lend an ear, let you vent, offer advice, or serve up some well-timed words of encouragement.

SparkTeams are online groups started by SparkPeople.com members who share common interests or goals. Teams have their own message-board forums, a place to talk about common interests and share tips with other members. Members who post on the community message boards or in SparkTeam forums tend to lose more weight than those who are not active in these areas.

There are SparkTeams from all over the world, grouped according to similar interests, goals, medical issues, or geography. In fact there are currently over 10,000 SparkTeams on SparkPeople.com, ranging from two members to hundreds of thousands. The groups include Dog Lovers, Dealing with Depression, Teachers Learning to Lose, SparkPeople's Weekend Survival Team, SparkGuy's 10-Minute Fitness Club, Rookie Runners, and Done Being the Fat Girl. There's something for everyone!

We have SparkTeams in cities across America as well as in other countries. Many of these people are starting to meet offline and do local activities and events together—even volunteer!

One of our priorities from the beginning was to build a powerfully positive online community for support, and we have spent countless hours fulfilling that dream. Spark-People members love our community and help protect it, making it a safe and supportive place for people to reach goals. We also have a special SparkTeam for longtime active members—the SparkPeople Community Team—which now numbers over 3,000 members around the world. This team helps welcome new members, lead other SparkTeams, and keep the community running smoothly.

We also have full-time employees, including personal trainers, registered dietitians, and motivation experts, who participate in the community and provide expertise. Each day I personally read messages from members as a way to stay motivated, and I have posted over 10,000 messages myself.

As a result of all of this, SparkPeople.com probably has the most active health-related online community in the world, with several million messages posted each month!

Even though our community is immense, you can find a SparkTeam that works for you. Once you find the right team or teams, this large community can feel like a small, tight-knit club. I've been so often touched by the support that people in the community give each other. Some people join and just log on and read other people's posts. Others end up posting and chatting daily, making some of the best friends they've ever had, sometimes with people across the world.

Our Emotional Eaters Team, with 157,000 members, is one of our largest. Leader SASSY describes what team members regularly do for each other:

> *Support, Compassion, Concern. That is what the EE team is all about. So many of us have dealt with this lifelong problem and realizing we are not alone, in itself, is a huge plus. We are there for each other every step of the way . . . We have welcomed new babies . . . new spouses . . . helped each other through the tragedies of death . . . suicide . . . serious illness*

*and organ transplant. We have a sub-team of the co-leaders that keeps all
leaders informed of anyone "in need" . . . as soon as we get a call . . . we
all take a moment to respond.*

Having community to support you and keep you motivated and accountable is one of the most crucial aspects of success, as our member FORME discovered. She started her journey at 225 pounds; she had dieted for ten years, but each time she ended up ten pounds heavier. Then she joined SparkPeople.

*Over the last year I have lost a little over 90 pounds. I no longer have
sleep apnea and I feel incredible. I have done things that I never thought
I would be able to do (run a 5K and 10K, bike the Cape 63 Miles, go rock
climbing)! What kept me going? My family. I started joining teams. I found
I really enjoyed talking with people who were in the same situation as me.
The biggest thing that I have gained over the last year is that I feel like I
am in control of my life!*

OVERCOME HURDLES

If you expect perfection, weight loss and healthy living can feel like a struggle. Faced with anything less than 100 percent success, you fall into guilty despair and revert to old habits. But at SparkPeople, we view healthy living as a journey, a process of learning. We know that life doesn't always pan out the way you planned and fate has a toolbox full of wrenches to throw into your path.

In the past ten years of working with millions of members, three hurdles have stood out to our experts. We're here to help you handle these real-life hurdles and prevent them from turning into downward spirals that can short-circuit your success.

Bounce Back from Setbacks

"Two steps forward, one step back" is usually a negative phrase used to describe someone who is having trouble making progress. But if you turn it around to "one step back, two steps forward," there's a whole new meaning. Instead of feeling guilty about a misstep, you can still come out ahead if you redouble your efforts and push forward.

Instead of expecting setbacks to go away and never recur, our most successful members acknowledge that they're an inevitable part of life, and they plan for them. They practice springing back up quickly whenever they take a fall, until it becomes a habit.

In our Secrets of Success survey, three times as many people who were "stuck" said they beat themselves up for having a bad day, as opposed to those who were successful and living healthy lifestyles. Treating yourself with kindness and compassion makes it more likely that you'll succeed. Beating yourself up is not only unproductive, it can trigger a downward spiral it may be hard to recover from.

Of all successful members, 84 percent said if they hit a setback in their pursuit of weight-loss or fitness goals, they simply acknowledged it and quickly moved on and got back on track. Literally none of our successful members said that they let setbacks derail their efforts.

We often hear members say, "Don't wait until January 1, or Monday, or summer, to get back on track after a setback! Do it today at 3:00 P.M., or tomorrow morning as soon as you get up." This can be the critical moment in determining whether you'll be successful and reach your goals. So many of us let setbacks send us on a downward spiral that can last for days, weeks, or even years. But once you learn how to deal with them, they become simply part of your journey, not permanent roadblocks.

Like our member FINALWIN:

> I've lost a lot of weight in the past, but whenever obstacles were in my way, I just gave up and gained again. I no longer see this as a diet; I no longer get really down on myself when I have a day of poor nutrition. I just move on, learn from it if I can, and make better choices. I'm 60 pounds lighter, more than halfway to my goal. For the first time in my entire life, I actually have the confidence that I will make it. I'm different now. Thank you SparkPeople, from the bottom of my (much healthier) heart!

What to Do When You're Stuck

We hear it all the time. You've changed your habits and lost weight steadily, but after a while, the progress halts. You've been stuck at the same weight for days, weeks, or even months. There's nothing more frustrating than trying your best, feeling like you are doing everything right, yet still being stalled.

There has been much debate about the concept of a weight-loss "plateau." Most experts now believe that plateaus are usually caused by straying from the details of your program and only sometimes caused by metabolic changes. It's true that there's often a tendency to become less accurate about how much you're actually eating and exercising once you get past the initial stage of being careful about everything. When you weigh less, you use less energy than you did when you were heavier, and since your body becomes naturally more efficient at repeated activities, you burn fewer calories. This is a good reason to increase your exercise intensity. Remember, too, that as you get closer to your final weight-loss goal, it 's natural to start losing less per week.

You should also keep in mind that even though the scale might have stopped moving, as long as you're still following your program, there still is magic happening in your body that hasn't shown up yet on the scale. Keep taking your measurements and noting your energy and happiness levels. Many of our successful members who stop focusing primarily on the scale end up being much happier and not letting it bother them when they are stuck. They just keep moving forward, knowing they are doing good things for their bodies and minds. And then often the scale starts moving again.

Is Emotional Eating a Problem?

Suppose you're eating plenty of veggies, your sleep is consistent, and you exercise so often that you're wearing out your gym shoes. It's hard to believe that something could still get in your way.

Something can, and often does: emotional eating.

Sometimes we eat for the strangest reasons. A bad day at work may culminate with a bag of barbeque chips on the couch. An argument may drive you to the fridge to calm down with ice cream. Emotional eating is possibly the number-one enemy of continued healthy living.

As you approach the completion of Week 3, it's time to consider the reasons behind possible pitfalls like these. You can—and should—eliminate emotional eating triggers so they no longer have a chance to sabotage your lifestyle and weight-loss success. While it's not always possible to pinpoint the exact root of these problems, you can take concrete steps to drive them out from the shadows.

1. Recognize the problem. You may be an emotional eater and not even realize it. Ask yourself a few questions: Do I often graze for no real reason, even though I'm not hungry? Have I found myself in front of an open fridge and not known why? Do I react to stress by opening my mouth and sticking a donut in it? Do I seem to gain weight when I'm going through hectic periods in my life?

2. Investigate and identify trigger times. Be aware of danger times and situations. Are weekends and holidays an emotional time for you? A visit with the in-laws? Talking with an ex? Do these times overlap with unhealthy eating episodes? The best way to figure this out is to carefully track your reasons for eating and anticipate problem triggers.

3. Ask why these triggers have power. The root of emotional eating often lies in large-scale issues. Are you going through a stressful period at work, at

home, or in your marriage? Have you had a recent failure that is crushing your self-esteem? Are you unhappy with your day-to-day life? Have you gone through a traumatic experience, such as a death, divorce, bankruptcy, or layoff? List everything in life that causes you stress. Learn to not worry about issues that are out of your control.

4.   Take it one trigger at a time. Write in your journal about how any of these larger life issues may be affecting your food choices and motivation. First, figure out how to recognize when the issue is about to trigger emotional eating and how to neutralize it. Then think about what steps you can take to keep the issue from taking hold of you. Focus on one issue at a time, and be patient and generous with yourself.

These steps can even help you start to solve some of the underlying major issues. Try hard to view the issues as challenges instead of stressors. Now that you are more confident about meeting challenges, you will be able to tackle these issues too!

That's what our member BVICTORIOUS did:

> *I rejoice over the triumphs—the gradual changing of my habits so that an apple is more appealing to me than a chocolate bar—wonder of wonders! I actually look forward to lacing up my running shoes to go for that walk or run. I love the feeling of fresh air filling my lungs and the joy that comes from the cool down of an exhilarating run. I love to dance, to move freely with joy! These are the things that encourage me. They are the strength that picks me up after that horrible weekend of indulging myself because I was lonely or bored. I keep on keeping on . . .*

SEE THE LIGHT

The world can be a beautiful place, full of possibilities and life. You can feel invincible and in control. But the world can also be a stressful, upsetting, confidence-crushing place. At times, it seems like even something as clear-cut as weight loss is harder than it needs to be. *Is it worth the trouble?* you ask yourself. *Why am I banging my head against the wall? Is it really doing any good?*

It absolutely is!

When life is difficult, you've got to take control of what you can. When confidence is low, that's exactly when you need to be at your healthiest, strongest, and most energetic. There's no better time to create your own little corner of sanity and positive feeling.

The best way to do that is to stick with those small healthy lifestyle goals. Drink your water, take your walk, log your food. Even if the results don't seem evident to you at this moment, it's your consistency, the fact that you can count on yourself, that will carry you through the tough times.

Remember, there will be good days and bad days, lazy days and discouraging ones. But there will also be days of revelation, of making breakthroughs and being proud of who you are becoming, days of wanting to climb on top of your success and reach for the stars, because you just know that anything is possible.

These are the days that make it all worthwhile, that let you deal with those other, not-so-great days. Once you know those bad days will be there, it's easier to accept them at face value and deal with them.

Don't let the world or your own doubts take away one of the most positive things you have going for yourself—your determination to create a healthier, more energetic, vibrant, and wonderful *you*.

Remember, I originally developed SparkPeople to help me conquer anxiety. When you have a setback or some issue that leads to emotional eating, it can be hard to "see the light." I know; I've been there. But stay strong, take heart, and keep taking one small positive step at a time.

WEEK 3 REVIEW

This week, you've become your own coach, learning an arsenal of strategies and skills that will benefit you for the rest of your life. One day at a time, you're gaining the sense of how it feels to be at the top of your game—full of energy, with a great attitude and a belief in yourself and your abilities. Now that you've learned to take two steps forward when faced with one step back, you can reach the stars!

CHAPTER 9

STAGE 4:
SPREAD THE SPARK

Have you ever watched a butterfly emerge from a cocoon, test its wings, and then fly off to begin its work pollinating plants and flowers? This metamorphosis is similar to what has been occurring inside you during these past weeks. Now that you are entering Week 4, you are becoming a different person—confident, stronger, and wiser. And with your new arsenal of skills, techniques, and habits, you're ready to spread your wings and take flight—inspiring others as you continue your transformed new life.

Just as a butterfly goes through four phases to become an adult, you have also traveled a journey to reach Week 4, the culmination of weeks of hard work.

In this crucial stage, we'll help you capitalize on your weight-loss success and put it to good use as a positive force. You'll be drawing on everything you've accomplished up till now to reach your goals and dreams and help others do the same.

In the Fast Break stage, when you were simply drinking eight cups of water or walking for ten minutes, this may not have seemed possible. But you're becoming a different person now. A new lifestyle, a new attitude, and a new supply of common-sense wisdom leave no doubt about it—you can do whatever you put your mind to. Go for it!

In this stage, you have four main purposes:

1. Help to "spark" others toward their own goals, which in turn helps you stay on track

2. Stay motivated to continue the healthy habits you've established

3. Learn how to transition from weight loss to weight maintenance

4. Pursue your new goals and dreams

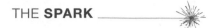

WEEK 4 ACTION STEPS

This week, we'll ask you to continue with the action steps from previous weeks as well as adding a few more.

1. Once you've read about spreading your spark to others, we'll ask you to choose one or more ways to do this in your own life.

2. You'll also set new goals that take you beyond this 28-day program—both in weight loss and fitness and beyond!

3. Finally, we'll ask you to make a SparkList of goals that you'd love to achieve in your lifetime. This fun activity will open your eyes to your life's potential and give you specific dreams to work toward that will keep you sparked.

SPREAD YOUR SPARK TO OTHERS

At SparkPeople we believe in the wisdom of the old epitaph: "What I gave, I have; what I spent, I had; what I kept, I lost."

When a match lights a candle, the flame doesn't shrink but grows. That's exactly what happens when you spread your spark. By inspiring and helping others, your program grows stronger.

SPREADING YOUR SPARK

- Keeps you engaged in your own lifestyle and connects you with others who share healthy goals

- Makes you accountable and more likely to uphold your own standards

- Positively impacts your own health—and if you're continuing to feel happy and healthy, you'll stick to your program all the more

- Makes you feel great. Thinking about others not only helps them, but takes your mind off yourself!

The crisscross effects for this week are unique; up until now, most of the effects have applied to different areas of *your* life. But this week is where the positive effects reach a new level—this is where your life positively impacts friends, family, co-workers, and your entire community! Just imagine millions of people living a sparked life, with crisscross effects flowing from one person to another all across the community in a great, positive network!

Helping Others Helps You

Of the successful SparkPeople members who lost 100 pounds or more, 88 percent said they try to encourage and support others who are on a weight loss or healthy lifestyle journey. Only 61 percent of those who were stuck helped other people. Further, when asked what was important to them, those who said that "helping other people/being a good friend, parent, kid, member of church or community" was most important had an edge on the general population when it came to many measures: they were more likely to reach their goals and lose more weight; they were much more likely to use motivational strategies such as giving themselves positive self-talk and connecting with other positive people; and they reported higher levels of happiness after doing the SparkPeople program. One hundred percent of these members said they actively spent time encouraging and supporting others.

Recent research has validated what we regularly see with our members—that lending a hand not only helps others, but helps us too. A study done at the University of Michigan showed that participants who were involved in regular volunteer work dramatically increased their life expectancy as well as boosting their vitality.[1] Another study reported that regular volunteer work induced a "helper's high," a warm, energetic, and calming feeling that contributed to mental and physical health.[2] More happiness and energy and less stress! These all will help fuel your own goals, in addition to making you feel great. And you'll discover how the benefits of healthy living extend far beyond the scale, into your living room, your office, even your neighborhood.

I can personally vouch for the satisfaction that comes from watching others become motivated and sparked. In my own life, this began when my co-worker Pat told me that I'd changed her life by inspiring her to pursue her own fitness and weight-loss goals—the comment that ultimately drove me to start SparkPeople in the first place.

In the years since, I've made over 10,000 message-board posts on SparkPeople.com. Each of these personal messages has helped me stay accountable to my own program. Talking to others about reaching their goals reminds me of my own and keeps me focused and excited.

And I see this same phenomenon occurring between members, as they gain meaning and accountability from cheering each other on. Without even realizing it, they're practicing leadership skills that will stand them in good stead in all areas of their lives.

Ways to Spread the Spark

Now that you're living a healthier lifestyle, you have the chance to use your new knowledge and leadership skills to serve as a positive force for others. I personally found it both exciting and a little scary to transition from being a follower in most social situations to becoming a leader. If you aren't used to taking the lead, just practice it one step at a time. By now you know that our formula works with just about any goal! If you are already a strong leader, great—now you have new skills from your healthy lifestyle adventure to share with others.

Since people are sometimes uncomfortable taking on public leadership roles, one way to practice this role is in the SparkPeople online community. There's no pressure and you can choose your level of participation. I've seen this work many times. For example, some members have told me that they were able to explore parts of their personality they never knew they had in the SparkPeople online community. They were then able to take those new skills into the "real world."

Try it yourself. You might be surprised at how much this helps you!

Spreading the spark is one of my favorite parts of SparkPeople; I've seen firsthand the magic it creates. When you positively impact another life, it leaves an imprint that can never be erased.

Members are always talking about how encouragement and advice from other members were the keys to their making a healthy lifestyle change. This community involvement, one person at a time helping another, is why SparkPeople is a movement that's making an impact on the world!

Set a Great Example

If you're uncomfortable proactively promoting weight loss and healthy lifestyle strategies with loved ones, friends, or colleagues, you can still help them by setting a great example. Simply living a fit and healthy life can impact others more than you know.

Here are some ideas for setting a healthy example:

- Take workout breaks at work. Proudly put on your walking shoes and go out for a workout at lunchtime.

- Hang photos in your office of walks, runs, or other active pursuits you've participated in.

- Walk or bicycle to work or to go shopping.

SOME WAYS TO SPREAD THE SPARK

- Start a walking club in your neighborhood, at school, or at work.

- Get five friends, family members, or co-workers to create a profile on SparkPeople.com. Encourage them to join an existing SparkTeam or even start their own!

- Volunteer to help with a charity race.

- Speak to a school class about fitness and nutrition.

- Volunteer at a local Meals on Wheels.

- Host a healthy-cooking dinner party for your block.

- Coach or assist a children's sports team.

- Start a tradition of cooking as a family.

- Plan an active vacation that includes hiking, biking, canoeing, or other physical activities.

- Help clean up a local park or playground.

- Volunteer at the local YMCA or community center.

- Explore a local mentoring program.

- Ask friends to donate seldom-used fitness equipment for charity.

- Donate healthy food to a local food drive.

- Trade healthy recipes with friends, family, and co-workers.

- Talk to a loved one about his or her health and why it's important to you that he or she stays healthy.

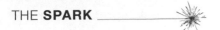

- Keep a variety of healthy foods or on your desk at work and in your kitchen.

- Order healthy foods when you're out at a restaurant with family or friends.

- Ask others to help you stay on track.

- Give lavish, positive praise for any healthy changes those around you have made.

- Choose a healthy restaurant or one that's within walking distance.

- Suggest a walking meeting (in which you solve a work issue while also burning calories) instead of a phone conference.

- Stock your kitchen with healthy cookbooks, leaving them where people can find them.

- Invite friends and family to play sports with you or accompany you when you work out.

Action Step: Choose one of these ways to spread your spark to others.

SPREAD THE SPARK IN YOUR OWN LIFE

Imagine that you're riding a bike in the Tour de France; you've ridden for three weeks, cycling over hills and vales, through rain and fog. Finally, exhausted but exhilarated, you reach the finish line. You're greeted by loved ones, flowers, and fanfare.

Now what? Do you dump your bike on the side of the road and forget about cycling for the rest of your life? Of course not! You relax, reenergize, then get back on your bike again and come up with a new destination.

It's the same with weight loss and healthy living. Now that your life has been sparked and you've developed an arsenal of strategies and healthy habits, you'll want to continue to use them as you look at broader vistas and reach for higher goals.

Week 4 is a great time to think ahead to how you'll keep yourself on track and build on your success. This week we'll give you tools and advice on how to do just that. Our members are always telling us that life really can be even better than they dreamed!

In fact, of successful members who lost weight and kept if off for at least six months, the majority kept their momentum at or close to the same level as during their early weight-loss program. They might switch to a higher calorie range for weight maintenance, but they continued their exercise, healthy foods, and pursuit of other goals.

We know that so much of success is about forward momentum. If you remain engaged in your healthy lifestyle, it will become a part of your daily life that naturally keeps you on track.

Be a Goal-Getter!

Of our successful members, 96 percent were actively working toward one or more goals. They all either had or had met weight loss goals, but they also had active fitness goals (81.5 percent), health- related goals (49 percent), and other life goals like financial, career, relationship, creative pursuits, and many more.

This secret to success is really important as you start out on your journey, but it has special significance here as you think about what's next. We know that using goal-setting techniques is key to weight loss, but we also believe it's essential to weight maintenance, as well as to reaching other life goals.

Remember, success begets more success! As you start reaching other important goals in life, you'll be even more excited about continuing your new healthy lifestyle. It's a wonderful upward spiral!

A New Definition of "Maintenance"

If the notion of maintenance seems dull to you, like something involving a car or appliance, we're here to change your mind. At SparkPeople, maintenance is a time of great excitement and promise—a time when you savor your progress, add new goals, revitalize your commitment, and spread your spark. You've already done much of the hard work—and now we're here to help you sustain it.

If you've met your weight-loss or fitness goals, congratulations! If you haven't met them yet, but made the switch from a diet to a healthy lifestyle, you should be equally thrilled. This change alone is one of the most important you'll ever make, and it will help you reach your ultimate weight and health goals and reach your fullest potential.

Our view of maintenance is unlike traditional diets, where people spend a limited period depriving themselves of calories, including most of the foods they love. Since they haven't developed a new lifestyle and are probably still secretly pining for these "bad" foods, they're likely to simply rush back to their old ways of eating once the diet is done. But with SparkPeople, you've developed a completely new lifestyle that can last a lifetime.

By developing an exercise program the right way, you have either hit your exercise tipping point or are getting close to it—and once you do, your healthy lifestyle will be a natural and fun part of your everyday life. Through our program, you've also probably developed a new appreciation for the varieties and pleasures of healthy foods. These new habits have increased the odds that you won't return to the same types and quantities of foods you used to eat. In Week 3, you learned what motivates you and how to stay motivated during setbacks, which makes you much less likely to slip back into old habits. You'll keep setting new goals, so that you will always be acting with purpose and reaching for new heights.

The most important difference between SparkPeople and other diets is that you now know that reaching your weight-loss goal is only one part of your entire life. In Week 4 of your program, you're still early in your healthy lifestyle adventure, but you have probably already discovered a newfound sense of confidence. Just imagine how you'll feel after you've kept up this momentum for the next three months, six months, or year. I can tell you from personal experience—and from witnessing the success of so many of our members—that you'll feel that anything is possible. And each goal you reach along the way will help you confirm this.

So, while our definition of maintenance may involve helping you keep your *weight* the same, your *life* will zoom ahead!

Secrets of Success of Maintainers

In our Secrets of Success survey, we took a look at the habits and behaviors of those who successfully met their weight-loss goals and had successfully maintained a healthy weight for at least six months (most, in fact, for over a year). What we found didn't surprise us. Those who maintained their weight loss (an average of 50 pounds!) remained very active in living a healthy lifestyle. The majority continue to eat within a healthy calorie range most days. Over 90 percent eat a healthy diet "most of the time" but most "don't worry too much" if they have a setback, they simply get back on track.

Successful maintainers also stay physically active. Eighty percent of them exercise three or more times a week and strength-train regularly. They also track their exercise at about the same rate as those still trying to lose weight. But they report a higher level of enjoyment of exercise once they get to this point in the program, perhaps illustrating that they have reached that "tipping point" and crossed the line into a positive, permanent healthy lifestyle.

Making the Transition from Weight Loss to Maintenance

How many calories should I be eating? How much exercise should I be doing? How do I prevent the weight from creeping back on?

These are common questions for those who have reached their weight-loss goal and now want to figure out how to maintain that loss. Most maintainers give themselves a weight range (usually five pounds or so) to stick to, since it can be tough to stay at exactly the same weight all the time because of natural fluctuations.

The following strategies will show you how to adjust your nutrition and fitness programs, as well as how to change your mindset from weight loss to weight maintenance.

- *Know your calorie needs for weight maintenance.* The first step toward weight maintenance is to calculate how many calories you can theoretically eat every day to maintain your present weight. A simple way to figure this out is to consult the Daily Calorie Needs chart in Chapter 7, the way you did when you first started. Only this time you won't have to account for weight loss, just your current weight and level of activity.

- *Work up (or down) to this calorie intake gradually.* Don't simply assume you can start eating at this maintenance level right away. You need to experiment a little until you figure out what your metabolism will allow. The best approach is to increase your daily calorie intake by 150 to 200 calories (from healthy food sources, of course) for one week and watch the effect this has on your weight. If you continue to lose weight, do the same thing again for another week. Continue doing this until you reach the estimated maintenance target you figured from the chart.

- *Exercise, exercise, exercise.* By far the most important factor in maintaining weight loss, according to the research, is a consistently high level of regular activity and exercise. Most likely, you will need to increase the intensity and/or duration of your exercise and other daily activity above what you did during the weight-loss phase so that your caloric expenditure remains a little higher than your maintenance-level calorie intake (as determined above).

For most people who are successful at weight maintenance, burning an additional 150 to 200 calories per day (above your normal daily exercise routine) seems to do the trick, though you may need to experiment a bit to find out what works for you. But make sure you *do not* reduce your calorie intake below the maintenance level in order to get out of doing more exercise or to "be safe." This could put you back in starvation mode. Rely on additional exercise, if necessary, to keep your weight stable.

Action Step: Set goals that will help you maintain your healthy weight and lifestyle.

MAINTENANCE CHECKS

Here are some good ways to stay on track:

- *Continue tracking your food.* You can do this daily, weekly, or a few times per month.

- *Continue tracking your exercise.* You can continue tracking your work-outs regularly, or choose to just track your exercise minutes for our online exercise competition, called SparkAmerica in the U.S. and SparkEarth around the world. This program inspires individuals, cities, states, and even entire countries to have a friendly competition with each other to see who can earn the most exercise minutes. You can help your team reach the top of the leaderboard!

- *Put it all together.* Come up with an inventory of what you've learned and the skills you've developed while losing weight. Think about how you can apply your knowledge and skills to maintain your weight—and to the next big challenge you decide to undertake.

SET YOUR SIGHTS HIGHER

Up until now you've been thinking in terms of a four-week program; now it's time to broaden your scope and look ahead at broader vistas. It's time to imagine how you can use the arsenal of strategies and healthy habits to reach even greater goals.

Our survey shows that members who maintain their weight continue to pursue active goals in fitness, health, finances, and relationships. Some of my favorite stories are from members who combine the techniques they've learned and use them in such areas as becoming a better parent or striving for a promotion at work.

What would you like to do next?

Now that you have either made a healthy lifestyle change or are on your way, you might be ready for other major breakthroughs. One of the best things about the Spark-People System is that improvements in one building block or cornerstone can lead to improvements in other building blocks or cornerstones. Go back and take a deeper look at the Focus cornerstone. I know that in my case, it wasn't until I had made a healthy lifestyle change that I started feeling more connected to myself and found it easier to figure out my real life's purpose.

Nine Ideas after Meeting Your Weight-Loss Goal

Here are several areas where you might set new goals:

1. *Let your career soar.* In a tight economy, good fitness and health are more important than ever. More confidence, energy, and brainpower will help whether you're in a job you love or you need the courage to move on to a new one. From making a presentation to handling conflict to acing a job interview, your new skills will make a difference. Think of a professional challenge that excites you and take the first step today.

2. *Be a hero to your kids.* Nobody is a perfect parent, but you've moved a little closer by getting in shape. Instead of collapsing at the end of a hard day or week, you might now be more inclined to help with homework or become involved in more spirited family activities like bike riding, canoeing, or sledding. The more you interact with your kids, the less they can interact with the TV. What a great example you've set!

3. *Lasso that financial beast.* Usually, when one part of life is out of control, the rest gets thrown into chaos too. By regaining control of your weight and health habits, you're gaining discipline and focus that can help you deal with finances. Whether you're getting out of debt or saving for retirement, your new goal-setting and tracking skills can make a mountain look like a molehill.

4. *Develop a new talent.* Painting, dancing, playing a musical instrument—these are artistic endeavors that appeal to many of us but are often bypassed in the rush of our busy lives. With SparkPeople, you've learned that building momentum is the key to overcoming doubt and fear. Hopefully, you've also learned that you can achieve anything you set your mind to. Time to go for it! This is a perfect goal for another weeklong, daily-action Fast Break.

5. *Wow your spouse or significant other.* You can't help but feel more romantic when you feel better about yourself. The positive attitude from weight loss has a real effect on those closest to you. Remember the SparkPeople concept that small things over time make a huge difference? Use it to consistently show your spouse how you feel with small gestures. It will quickly become a regular—and welcome—habit.

6. *Become a student again.* Going back to school can be intimidating. For people already crunched for time, it can seem impossible. But as your weight-loss plan is proving, with planning and organization—not to mention your newfound energy levels—anything is possible. When you're eating healthy and exercising, your memory is sharper, making studying and learning a snap—even conjugating those French verbs. Of course, you can also choose to expand your vistas in other ways.

7. *Start your own business.* Long hours, potential stress, a nonstop schedule: these are the rewards of striking out on your own. But so are freedom, excitement, and a life-changing experience. To brave this path, you'll need to be at the top of your game. That means loads of energy, a great attitude, and a belief in yourself and your abilities. Being in shape makes this all the more possible.

8. *Rediscover your social life.* Did spontaneity disappear while your waistline grew? Now that you lead a healthier and more active life, bring your friends along for the ride. Plan fun activities, join a team, keep a journal of all the high points (for later motivation), and enjoy yourself. This is where all your hard work can pay off.

9. *Keep improving your health and fitness.* Once you've lost your goal weight, does that mean the job is done, so you can go back to your old habits and cruise on through? Of course not. This is a great opportunity to build even more healthy habits that help you consistently feel and look a little better every day. Maybe now you'd like to go to the next level and get involved in a sport you love! Maybe it's time to turn your newfound love of walking into participating in a charity walk, or go from jogging on your treadmill to running a 5K, a half-marathon, or more!

Four Ways to Keep Going for the Long Haul

Just as you wouldn't take a long trip without planning your route and watching the road signs, you shouldn't expect to accomplish new long-term goals without planning your journey and monitoring your progress.

Here are four creative ways to monitor your progress as you reach for new dreams:

1. *Buy or create a goal calendar.* This can be large enough to hang or small enough to carry with you. Mark the daily progress you make toward your

goals, and briefly note problems, challenges, and successes that you experience. You can also chart higher-level goals on a monthly, quarterly, or even yearly basis.

2. *E-mail your own encouragement.* Send yourself a daily e-mail reviewing how you did yesterday and what you plan to do today. You can do this at the end of each day or even at the beginning of your day. Just seeing the current e-mail in your inbox—or even glancing over it once or twice a day—is a powerful reminder that you want to accomplish something worthwhile.

3. *Journal.* Keeping a daily journal of your progress is a great way to review your challenges and successes. Include how you do and how you feel about your progress. Remember, if this is your main tracking tool, you must do it every day for it to be effective.

4. *Report to a buddy.* Find a friend you can talk with briefly—daily or weekly, online or by phone—to help track your progress in tackling your goals. Make sure you choose a positive person who's willing to be helpful and encouraging. Better yet, find someone who has goals of his or her own and can use your input in track his or her progress.

Here's one of our favorite stories by a SparkPeople member, a writer who admitted on her SparkPage that she hadn't found luck in either writing or losing weight. But once she joined SparkPeople, she not only lost weight but also landed a significant two-book deal from a major publisher and found herself traveling through Italy, doing the work of her dreams.

> *I have vivid memories of walking up and down the hills around my California home as part of my Spark Program and carrying a tape recorder because the exercise often led to breakthroughs in my writing. Some of the best lines in my book The Book of Unholy Mischief came to me while I was hiking through orange groves.*
>
> *And then walking all over Venice ON CAMERA and hiking in the Himalayas—all of it would have been impossible without my Spark training. Not to mention the discipline learned from tracking my food and making time for my walks.*
>
> *I found SparkPeople through a writer friend in NY. She lost 188 pounds, and I asked her what she would recommend for a 20-pound loss. She said SparkPeople was the best program out there, and it is . . . I have made real, honest-to-God friends on SparkPeople. I've never met them in person but I feel I've known them forever. You have touched millions of lives.*

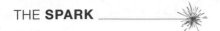

Elle's story shows how you can use your healthy lifestyle as a springboard to reach other amazing goals. Breakthroughs like this can change the course of your entire life. We want to help you make this happen!

Action Step: Think about additional goals you might want to pursue and make a plan to take steps toward reaching them.

YOUR SPARKLIST

Dare to dream! One thing you've learned is that reaching goals is infectious. Once you reach one, you'll want to reach more. Here's an exercise that captures that spirit.

We challenge you to list 50 to 100 things you'd like to do in your lifetime. These can be big goals or small, for important causes or pure pleasure. This fun exercise may help you learn about yourself and figure out the long-term goals you want to set.

Here are some possible categories for your top 50 to 100:

- Places you'd like to visit and why
- Skills you'd like to learn
- Experiences you'd like to have
- Fun things you'd like to do
- Books you'd like to read
- Achievements you'd like to reach

Action Step: Are you ready? Start making your SparkList!

IN CLOSING

At SparkPeople, we believe (as writer Paulo Coehlo does) that "when we strive to become better than we are, everything around us becomes better, too."

Now that you have completed the 28-day program, you have earned the reward you set in the Fast Break—congratulations!

CONCLUSION

We recently hosted the first SparkPeople convention in San Diego. Hundreds of members—from moms to Navy submarine officers—joined together to celebrate and testify to the way SparkPeople has changed their lives.

It was incredible to feel the exuberance and power of so many members gathered together. And it was personally gratifying and awe-inspiring to realize that a program I devised so many years ago to help my own anxiety has grown to impact so many others. Now I'm just a small part of something special. Looking out at the crowds of people streaming together, smiling, and sharing inspiring stories was humbling, a milestone of satisfaction and pride.

The convention reinforced one of the most essential aspects of our program—authenticity. Our program is about real people like you who are genuinely transforming themselves.

Leah from San Diego was one member who stood out. She's lost 62 pounds on SparkPeople, but that was just the beginning. Now she's also the leader of our San Diego SparkTeam and regularly gets her team together for activities. Her leadership skills were obvious from the moment I met her. She said, "I used to be a follower. Because of Spark-People I've learned to become a leader. I want the members of my team to succeed and become leaders themselves."

Soon after, Leah was on stage in front of hundreds of people telling others, "If I can do it, you can do it, too!"

At the convention, I also met Elle Newmark, the member who landed a major book deal as part of her SparkPeople adventure and embarked on an exciting trip to Italy, the setting of her book. But she didn't stop there, as she told us:

> I just spent a month in India, researching my next book. That little hill in California near my home is laughable compared to the Himalayas where life is entirely vertical. I spent almost two weeks at altitudes between 6,000 and 8,000, and was able to see and do everything. This enhanced physical ability creates a sense of well-being, self-sufficiency, and plain old power that

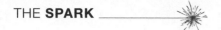

is priceless. I am 62 years old and I feel like the world is mine for the taking. I can go places and do things that would have been unthinkable 3 years ago. My SparkPeople experience wasn't a dream come true, I never even dreamed this. All that happened to me was beyond what I ever dreamed.

This is my parting hope for you—that you will use your new, healthy lifestyle to reach goals and enjoy experiences you may never even have imagined. If you ever need help along the way, you now know where you can find a source of amazing support. We're here for you, all along the way.

Welcome to your sparked life!

SPARKPEOPLE MIX-AND-MATCH MEALS

Cooking at home is a great way to keep on track. You know what's going into your food and are better able to control calories and fat. However, many of us rely on restaurants and on processed foods, which are full of salt, fat, and calories.

Cooking may be a lost art, but it's one that's easy to learn. We've created a step-by-step meal system that helps you develop your own recipes or menu combinations—and eventually cook without any recipes at all. Consider this meal system your safety net. Once you know how much food you should be eating and what kinds of foods to eat regularly, you can get more creative and whip up healthful meals on your own.

In the pages that follow, you'll find mix-and-match charts that outline what to eat in each food group for each meal. For breakfast, we'll show you how to combine milk, fruit, carbs, and protein to create a well-balanced, healthy meal. For lunch, we break down salads and sandwiches into their nutritional components to give you delicious options that come in under 400 calories. For dinner, we look at how to combine carbs, vegetables, proteins, and starches to create easy, nutritious meals.

Following each meal—breakfast, lunch, and dinner—you'll find two samples of recipes that have been made by our SparkPeople members. These are just examples of the kinds of things you can make by picking and choosing from the mix-and-match charts. You can find thousands more of these recipes at Recipes.SparkPeople.com.

And after showing just how easy mixing and matching can be, we outline two complete days' worth of scrumptious, healthy food to help you begin your journey.

The charts teach you what foods you should be eating, the recipes show you how to put them together, and the meal plans show you how to fit them into your daily life. So let's get started!

MIX-AND-MATCH MEAL CHARTS

Any of these combinations will result in meals that are no more than 400 calories each, and many combinations come closer to 300 calories. Our guidelines for breakfasts and lunches give amounts for one serving; our dinner suggestions serve four, which means you can either have nutritious leftovers for the next day or serve your entire family a tasty, healthful dinner.

Breakfast

Breakfast is the most important meal of the day, and for good reason. Studies show that people who eat a well-balanced breakfast consume fewer calories throughout the day and rev up their metabolisms. Starting the day with both carbohydrates and lean protein can help lessen cravings and hunger the rest of the day. We've compiled breakfasts that are so easy, even the most time-strapped of us can make time for a healthy morning meal.

The calories below are for one serving size, but feel free to add a second serving if you have room in your calorie budget.

While you might want to skimp on calories and fat at breakfast and "bank" them for the rest of the day, resist the urge. Follow the old adage: "Eat like a king at breakfast, a prince at lunch, and a pauper at dinner."

Choose one serving from each category to create a nutritious breakfast.

Milk: Include a glass of skim milk or calcium-fortified nondairy milk, a serving of fruit, and a mix of protein and carbs for breakfast each day.

Milk (8-oz servings)	Calories	Fat (g)
Almond milk*	50	2.5
Rice milk*	110	2.5
Skim milk	90	0
Soy milk*	100	4

Choose a calcium-fortified version.

Fruit: Though vegetables get most of the attention for their antioxidant power, fruits should not be absent from a healthy diet. Aim to get at least two of your five (or more) servings of produce from fruit each day. Choose whole fruit over fruit juice whenever possible for added fiber and nutrients.

A serving of fresh or frozen fruit is a half-cup, which is about the size of a billiard ball. Choose half an apple, pear, orange, or banana or a half-cup of berries, melon, or tropical fruit. A serving of juice is six ounces, about half of a soda can.

Fruit	Serving size	Calories
Apple	½ large	41
Banana	½ large	63
Blueberries	½ c	41
Cranberries (dried)	2 T	46
Grapes	½ c	48
Mango	½ c	54
Melon	½ c	32
Orange	½ large	44
Pear	½ large	62
Pineapple (fresh)	½ c	60
Raisins	2 T	55
Raspberries	½ c	30
Strawberries	½ c	23

Carbohydrates: Carbs have gotten a bad rap in recent years, but they should be a part of a healthy meal, especially breakfast. Complex carbohydrates (whole grains) take a while to absorb, resulting in steady blood sugar levels, which allow you to feel "full" longer and give you lasting energy. Whole grains are also packed with nutrients and fiber.

Aim for 6 to 11 servings of grains daily. A serving of grains is equal to one ounce of bread (one small slice, ½ bagel, ½ bun), about the size of a plastic CD case. A serving of cooked grains or dry cereal is ½ cup, about the size of a billiard ball.

Carbs	Serving size	Calories	Fat (g)
Bread (whole wheat)	1 slice	80	1
English muffin (whole wheat)	1 muffin	120	1
Flake cereal (whole grain)	½ c	70	0.5
Granola (low-fat)	¼ c	105	1.5
Granola bar	1 bar	120	5
Grape-Nuts	¼ c	104	0.5
Grits	½ c	83	0.5
Mini-bagel (whole wheat)	1 mini	110	1
Oats (dry)	½ c	148	2.5
Pancakes (whole wheat)	1, 4" pancake	92	3

Shredded wheat	½ c	83	0.5
Toaster waffle (whole wheat)	1 waffle	70	1
Tortilla (whole wheat)	1, 8" tortilla	130	3

Protein: Protein helps keep you fuller longer and takes longer to digest than vegetables and carbs. Meat, cheese, nuts, and nut butters all provide protein. Aim for two or three servings daily.

Protein	Serving size	Calories	Fat (g)
Almonds	½ oz	82	7
American cheese	1 oz	60	4.5
Canadian bacon	2 slices	86	4
Cheddar cheese (low fat)	1 oz	50	2
Cottage cheese (1% milkfat)	4 oz	81	1
Cheese (Laughing Cow)	1 wedge	50	4
Egg (whites)	¼ c	25	0
Egg (whole)	1 scrambled or poached	74	5
Nut butter	1 T	105	8
Sunflower seeds (no salt)	½ oz	83	7
Yogurt (flavored, low fat)	4 oz	99	1
Yogurt (plain, low fat)	4 oz	71	2

Extras: Complete your breakfast with one of these extras, if you have room in your calorie budget for the day.

Extra	Serving size	Calories	Fat (g)
All-fruit spread	1 T	40	0
Chocolate syrup	1 T	50	0
Cinnamon	½ t	6	0
Cream cheese (light)	1 oz	74	7
Flaxseed (ground)	1 T	30	2
Honey	½ T	32	0
Maple syrup (real)	1 T	52	0
Margarine	1 t	34	4
Salsa	¼ c	18	0
Sugar	1 t	16	0
Turkey bacon	2 slices	34	3

FRUITY OATMEAL

Cook:
  ½ c dry oats according to package directions
  (148 calories, 2.5 g fat)

Remove from heat and top with:
  ½ large pear, chopped (62 calories)
  ½ oz chopped almonds (82 calories, 7 g fat)
  1 T real maple syrup (52 calories)

Serve with:
  1 c skim milk (90 calories)

Total: 434 calories, 9.5 g fat

BREAKFAST ON THE RUN

No time for breakfast? Not so fast. A smoothie in a to-go cup,
with a granola bar on the side, is great for busy commuters.
You can substitute your favorite fruit, nut butter, or milk
for the soy milk here.

Blend:
  1 c soy milk (100 calories, 4 g fat)
  ½ c frozen mango chunks (54 calories)
  1 T peanut butter (105 calories, 8 g fat)
  1 T ground flaxseed (30 calories, 2 g fat)
  4 ice cubes

Eat with:
  1 low-fat granola bar (120 calories, 5 g fat)

Total: 409 calories, 19 g fat

Lunch

Salads and sandwiches are easy, affordable lunches. We've created two charts to help you expand your palate while keeping your wallet and stomach full. Our meal suggestions are healthful and bursting with fruits and vegetables so you get to eat more food for fewer calories.

Salads

Salads are a great way to get in your five-a-day servings of fruits and vegetables (or even more). Follow our instructions to create a filling salad with a maximum of 400 calories. We even leave room for a couple of higher-calorie "treat" items in your salad!

Greens: Start with a heaping bowl of dark, leafy greens. Try to bypass iceberg for sturdier, darker greens, which pack more of a nutritional punch. You'll get antioxidants, vitamins, and fiber.

Choose at least two of the greens below (enough to make up about 40 calories).

Salad base	Serving size	Calories
Arugula	2 c	10
Baby greens (mixed)	2 c	30
Cabbage (shredded)	2 c	35
Iceberg	2 c	15
Romaine	2 c	16
Spinach	2 c	14

Protein: Protein helps keep us fuller longer and takes longer to digest. Beans, cheese, meat, and seafood are all good lean proteins to include in salads. Pick any combination of cheese, meat, seafood, and beans to add about 225 calories to your salad.

Protein	Serving size	Calories	Fat (g)
Black beans	½ c	114	0.5
Bleu cheese	2 T	60	5
Cheddar cheese (low fat)	1 oz	49	2
Chicken (grilled)	3 oz	94	1
Chickpeas	½ c	143	1
Cottage cheese (1% milkfat)	4 oz	82	1
Deli turkey, cut in strips	3 oz	90	1
Egg (hard boiled)	1 whole	74	5

Feta cheese (low fat)	1 oz	60	4
Flank steak	3 oz	131	6
Goat cheese (soft)	1 oz	76	6
Kidney beans	½ c	109	0.5
Mozzarella cheese (part skim)	1 oz	72	4.5
Parmesan cheese	2 T	46	3
Salmon fillet	3 oz	127	4
Shrimp	3 oz	90	1.5
Swiss cheese (low fat)	1 oz	90	6

Fruits and Vegetables: Fruits and vegetables add flavor and texture to a salad for very few calories. Both vegetables and fruit offer fiber, vitamins, and antioxidants, which help fight disease and keep our bodies healthy.

Mix and match fruits and vegetables to equal about 90 calories. Aim for at least three or four vegetables in different colors.

Fruit/vegetable	Serving size	Calories
Asparagus	½ c	26
Beets	½ c	29
Bell peppers	½ c	20
Blueberries	½ c	20
Broccoli	½ c	12
Cauliflower	½ c	13
Celery	½ c	10
Cucumbers	½ c	7
Grapes	½ c	48
Mushrooms	½ c	15
Onions	½ c	14
Peas	¼ c	28
Radishes	½ c	9
Raspberries	½ c	30
Red cabbage (shredded)	½ c	14
Roasted red peppers*	½ c	25
Strawberries	½ c	23
Sun-dried tomatoes*	¼ c	35
Squash	½ c	14
Tomatoes	½ c	25

* Not packed in oil

Salad Dressing: Dressings help flavors mix and add another layer of flavor to salads. Fight the urge to drown your salad in dressing. Measure out two tablespoons, about the size of a ping-pong ball. Dip the tines of your fork in the dressing before each bite or drizzle on just a bit of dressing to start.

We chose dressings that add fewer than 60 calories per serving.

Dressing	Serving size	Calories	Fat (g)
Bleu cheese (low fat)	2 T	45	2
Caesar (low fat)	2 T	50	2
French (low fat)	2 T	44	2
Italian (low fat)	2 T	35	2
Lemon juice	2 T	6	0
Olive oil	2 T	60	7
Ranch (low fat)	1 T	40	2
Raspberry vinaigrette (low fat)	2 T	35	2
Salsa	½ c	36	0
Sour cream (low fat)	2 T	20	2
Vinegar	2 T	7	0

Extras: If you have the room in your calorie budget for the day, add one of these "treats" to your salad. They can take your salad over the 400-calorie mark, so don't try to skimp on greens or vegetables to fit them in—calculate these calories in addition to whatever your salad contains. Tip: crumble, slice, or chop high-calorie salad items to stretch their flavor throughout your salad.

Treat	Serving size	Calories	Fat (g)
Almonds	½ oz	82	7
Avocado	¼ fruit	72	7
Bacon (crumbled)	1 slice	37	3
Bread/roll (whole grain)	1 slice/roll	80	1.5
Capers	2 T	4	0
Cranberries (dried)	¼ c	47	0
Croutons (baked, whole grain)	1/2 oz	58	1
Olives	6 jumbo	40	3
Raisins	2 T	55	0
Sunflower seeds	½ oz	83	7
Tortilla chips (baked)	1 oz	110	2
Walnuts	½ oz	93	9

Sandwiches

It's noon, and you're about to open your brown bag. So why aren't you excited? Maybe to you, the word "sandwich" evokes the doldrums—or maybe it conjures the image of a jaw-breaking, gut-busting, fat-laden monstrosity piled high with greasy meats, heavy cheeses, and gloppy mayonnaise. Think again!

It's time to go beyond the PB&J and the ham and Swiss. Sandwich rules are simple: Bread or a similar product with your choice of ingredients in between. The rest is up to you! Here's a list of ingredients to get you started. Mix and match your favorites or try something new.

Any sandwich you put together using these ingredient suggestions, with bread, protein, cheese, vegetable, and a couple of condiments, should add up to about 400 calories.

Bread: Start with a base for your sandwich. Choose whole grains for added fiber. Tip: leave off one slice of bread for an open-faced sandwich and save up to 85 calories.

Bread	Serving size	Calories	Fat (g)
Baguette (multigrain)	1, 3" piece	140	1.5
Bun (whole wheat)	1 bun	140	2
Mixed-grain bread	2 slices	130	2
Pita (whole wheat)	1, 6" pita	170	1.5
Pumpernickel bread	2 slices	130	1.5
Rye bread	2 slices	166	2
Sprouted-grain bread	2 slices	160	1
Tortilla (wheat or corn)	1, 8" tortilla	130	3
Whole-wheat bread	2 slices	160	2

Protein: Protein helps keep you fuller longer and takes longer to digest than vegetables and carbs. Meat, cheese, and nut butters all provide protein. Choose lean, low-sodium deli meats.

Protein	Serving size	Calories	Fat (g)
Chicken (grilled)	3 oz	94	1
Egg	1 whole	74	5
Ham	3 oz	90	2
Hummus	¼ c	104	6
Nut butter	1 T	105	8
Roast beef	2 oz	100	2
Salmon fillet	2 oz	85	3
Tofu (broiled)	2 oz	92	6

Tuna (in water)	3 oz	99	1
Turkey	3 oz	90	1
Turkey bacon	2 slices	34	3

Because most sandwiches have meat and cheese, we've reduced the serving size of the cheese to save calories. Tip: skip the meat if you want a full serving of cheese.

Cheese	Serving size	Calories	Fat (g)
American	½ oz slice	30	2
Bleu	½ oz slice	30	2.5
Cheddar (low fat)	½ oz slice	25	1
Cream cheese (light)	½ oz	37	3
Feta (low fat)	½ oz	30	2
Goat cheese (soft)	½ oz	37	3
Gouda	½ oz slice	51	4
Mozzarella (part skim)	½ oz slice	36	2
Swiss (low fat)	½ oz slice	45	3

Vegetables: Vegetables are generally low in calories but pack quite the nutritional punch. Pile on the raw veggies to get an array of vitamins and antioxidants, plus fiber. Tip: use peppers, onions, and other vegetables to add flavor to your sandwich for few calories.

Vegetable	Serving size	Calories
Banana peppers	2 T	4
Basil leaves	4 leaves	1
Bell peppers	¼ c	10
Carrot slices	½ carrot	13
Celery (chopped)	½ c	10
Cucumbers	6 slices	3
Onions	1 thick slice	14
Pickles	6 slices	8
Romaine lettuce	1 large leaf	1.5
Spinach	½ c	3.5
Sprouts	¼ c	2
Tomatoes	3 slices	13
Zucchini slices	¼ c	7

Condiments: Condiments should not be the focus of the sandwich. Instead of piling on gloppy, creamy sauces, use mustards, ketchup, or other low-calorie condiments and sauces to enhance the flavor of your sandwich. Tip: mash roasted garlic into a paste and spread it on for extra flavor.

Condiment	Serving size	Calories	Fat (g)
All-fruit spread	1 T	42	0
Avocado, mashed	2 T	48	4
Barbecue sauce	1 T	40	0
Garlic (roasted)	2 cloves	10	0
Honey mustard	1 T	30	0
Ketchup	1 T	15	0
Mayo (low fat)	1 T	50	5
Mustard	1 T	10	0
Pesto	1 t	24	2
Ranch dressing (low fat)	1 T	40	2
Salsa	2 T	10	0
Tomato sauce	1 T	5	0
Vinaigrette (low fat)	1 t	8	1

Some sandwich strategies to lighten your load:

- Limit yourself to one creamy or higher-fat item. Either cheese or mayo. Either bacon or avocado. Not both.

- Try smoked cheese (cheddar, mozzarella, provolone, and Gouda all come in smoked varieties) to add another level of flavor to your sandwich.

- Make your own mayo substitute. Mix low-fat or fat-free yogurt (try Greek-style) with your favorite herb or spice blend. Be creative—try curry powder, your favorite grill rub, dried herbs like dill or tarragon, spicy mustard, or even your favorite jam. Spread this on your bread.

- Shrink your sandwich. Make it with a couple of mini-pitas or mini-bagels instead of full-size bread.

- Go halvsies. Split a sandwich with a friend and add a side salad or a piece of fruit.

- Ditch the cheese. There's plenty of flavor in your sandwich already.

- Go topless. Use only one slice of bread, then pile on the toppings.

- If you're toasting your bread, don't butter or oil it first. Use a quick spritz of nonstick cooking spray.

- Think of the vegetables as a main ingredient, not an afterthought. Add an extra serving! Berries, grilled onions, spinach, tomatoes, or roasted peppers are great on grilled cheese. Pile extra lettuce or spinach on any sandwich.

- Use mustard, vinegar, or chutneys instead of creamy condiments.

- Think beyond ketchup, mustard, and mayo. Slather some salad dressing, a marinade, or even your favorite sauce or salsa on your bread.

- Love bleu cheese but not the fat and calories? Mix a small amount with fat-free plain yogurt to spread out that strong flavor.

SETTING THE (SALAD) BAR HIGH

Toss:
   2 c mixed baby greens (30 calories)
   2 c Romaine lettuce, chopped (16 calories)

Top with:
   1 hard-boiled egg, sliced (74 calories, 5 g fat)
   4 oz light (1% milkfat) cottage cheese (82 calories, 1 g fat)
   ½ c sliced mushrooms (15 calories)
   ½ c cherry tomatoes (25 calories)
   ½ c celery, diced (10 calories)
   ½ c roasted red peppers, chopped (25 calories)

Drizzle on:
   2 T low-fat Italian dressing (35 calories, 2 g fat)

Serve with:
   1 slice whole-grain bread (80 calories, 1.5 g fat)

Total: 392 calories, 9.5 g fat

ITALIAN TURKEY-PESTO SANDWICH

Toast:
   2 slices mixed-grain bread (130 calories, 2 g fat)

Top with:
   3 oz lean, low-sodium deli turkey (90 calories, 1 g fat)
   ½ oz part skim mozzarella (36 calories, 2 g fat)
   3 slices tomato (13 calories)
   ¼ c bell pepper rings (10 calories)
   4 basil leaves (1 calorie)

Slather on:
   2 cloves roasted garlic (10 calories)
   1 t pesto (24 calories, 2 g fat)

Serve with:
   ½ large banana (63 calories)
   1 c water

Total: 377 calories, 5 g fat

Dinner

In these tables, we've listed a "total" amount of each ingredient to yield four individual servings. To make more or fewer portions, just change the total you start with.

Protein: A serving of meat, fish, or tofu should be about the size of a deck of cards or the palm of your hand (two to three ounces cooked). A pound of meat, poultry, or seafood yields about 12 ounces cooked. Trim any visible fat from meat before cooking, and choose the leanest cuts possible.

Sauté, bake, or broil, using nonstick cooking spray if necessary, one of the following meats and proteins.

Protein	Total to serve 4 (raw)	Serving size (cooked)	Calories	Fat (g)
Beef (ground, 96% lean)	16 oz	3 oz	150	4.5
Black beans*	2 c	½ c	114	0.5
Chicken breast	16 oz	3 oz	94	1
Chickpeas*	2 c	1½ c	143	1
Eggs	4 eggs	1 egg	74	5
Lentils*	2 c	½ c	115	0.5
Salmon	16 oz	3 oz	127	4
Shrimp	16 oz	3 oz	90	1.5
Tofu	2 c	½ c	137	8
Tuna	16 oz	3 oz	127	4
Turkey cutlets	16 oz	3 oz	82	2
Veggie burgers	4 patties	1 patty	150	2.5
White fish**	16 oz	3 oz	68	1

*Drain and rinse canned beans, then add seasonings and heat.
**Tilapia, cod, pollock, and halibut are all varieties of fish that have white flesh and can be used interchangeably.

Vegetables: A serving of cooked vegetables is ½ cup, about the size of a billiard ball. A serving of greens or raw vegetables is one cup, about the size of a baseball when raw. Be sure to eat a variety of vegetables in all colors each day. You can substitute a serving of fruit for a serving of vegetables, but note that fruit is often more caloric, so adjust accordingly. While the protein is cooking, chop, then sauté, steam, or microwave two of these vegetables:

Vegetable	Total to Serve 4	Serving size	Calories
Asparagus	2 c	½ c	15
Bell peppers	1 large	¼ pepper	13
Broccoli	2 c	½ c	12
Brussels sprouts	2 c	½ c	28
Carrots	2 c	½ c	26
Cauliflower	2 c	½ c	13
Collards (or other greens)	4 c	1 c	11

Eggplant	2 c	½ c	11
Green beans	2 c	½ c	17
Mushrooms	2 c	½ c	8
Onion	1 large	¼ onion	14
Peas	2 c	½ c	55
Tomatoes	4 fresh or 2 c canned	1 tomato or ½ c canned	26
Spinach	4 c	1 c	7
Winter squash	2 c	½ c	41
Zucchini (or other squash)	2 c	½ c	14

Carbohydrates: Whole-grain carbs are an important part of a healthy meal plan. While we should get 6 to 11 servings of grains daily, we tend to eat oversize portions. A serving of bread is one ounce, about the size of a plastic CD case. A serving of cooked grains or potatoes is ½ cup, about the size of a billiard ball.

Add one of these whole-grain carbs to your recipe or as a side dish:

Carbohydrates	Total to Serve 4	Serving size	Calories	Fat (g)
Bread or rolls (whole wheat)	4 slices or rolls	1 slice or roll	80	1.5
Couscous*	2 c cooked (1 c dry)	½ c	88	0
Pasta (whole grain)**	4 oz	¼ c	95	0
Potatoes (baked, boiled, or roasted)	2 c (about 2 small)	½ c	64	0
Rice (brown)*	2 c cooked (1 c dry)	½ c	108	1
Sweet potatoes (baked)	2 c (2 medium)	½ c	70	0

Cook grains with a 2:1 ratio of water or low-sodium broth to grains.
*** We cut the serving size of the pasta to keep the meal under 400 calories. If you have room in your calorie budget for the day, you may eat a larger serving.*

Additional Seasonings: Think beyond salt and pepper. Seasonings, herbs, and spices add negligible calories and no fat. Add dried seasonings (plus garlic, peppers, and onion if you're using them) while cooking the protein; add chopped fresh herbs at the end of cooking.

Experiment with a few spice blends and add your favorite herbs and spices liberally. If you use seasoning blends from the supermarket, be sure to choose salt-free varieties.

Herb/spice	Amount
Basil (dried or fresh)	2 T dried or handful fresh
Chili flakes	½ t (to taste)
Cilantro (fresh)	¼ c
Coriander	1 T
Cumin	2 T
Curry	1 T
Dill (dried)	1 T
Ginger (fresh, grated)	1"
Mint (dried or fresh)	1 T dried or handful fresh
Oregano (dried)	1 t
Paprika (smoked)	1 T
Parsley (fresh)	handful
Poultry seasoning	2 T
Rosemary (dried)	1 T
Taco seasoning*	3 T
Tarragon (dried)	1 T
Thyme (dried)	½ T

Forget the sodium-laden taco spice packets. Make home-made, salt-free taco seasoning: mix 1 tablespoon cumin, 1 tablespoon chili powder, and 1 teaspoon paprika. Add more or less of any spice to taste.

Sauces: Food can be healthful and flavorful without adding excess fat and calories. We've created a few low-calorie and low-fat sauce and seasoning combinations to help rescue you from mealtime boredom. Once your protein is cooked, mix in one of these sauces. Choose low-fat, low-sodium sauces whenever possible.

Sauce	Total to Serve 4	Serving size	Calories	Fat (g)
Barbecue sauce**	½ c	2 T	52	0
Broth (low sodium)	½ c	2 T	5	0
Honey mustard	¼ c	1 T	30	0
Ketchup	½ c	2 T	15	0
Lemon juice/zest	2 lemons	½ lemon	6	0
Orange juice	½ c	2 T	14	0
Parmesan cheese	¼ c	1 T	23	1.5

Ranch dressing (low fat)	¼ c	1 T	40	2
Salsa	2 c	½ c	35	0
Sour cream (light)	¼ c	1 T	20	0
Soy sauce	2 T	½ T	4	0
Tomato sauce	2 c	½ c	40	0.5
White wine*	½ c	2 T	20	0

Turn heat on high briefly to cook off alcohol.

**Make your own quick barbecue glaze. Mince three cloves of garlic, then mix with 4 teaspoons brown sugar, 2 tablespoons cider vinegar, and ½ cup no-salt-added tomato paste. This will be thick; use a bit of water to reach desired consistency. Season to taste and spread on meat, fish, or tofu before cooking. It pairs well with the homemade taco seasoning above.*

Extras: Add a glass of milk and a serving of fruit to round out your meal.

CREAMY DILL CHICKEN WITH GREEN BEANS AND CARROTS (SERVES 4)

16 oz chicken breasts, divided into four portions
2 c frozen green beans
2 c frozen carrots
4 whole-grain dinner rolls
1 T fresh dill, chopped
¼ c light sour cream
salt and pepper

Optional: lemon wedges, garlic powder, or 1 clove minced garlic

Preparation:

Preheat broiler and place rack six inches from the source of heat. Trim visible fat from chicken, then place on broiling pan or baking sheet. Broil chicken for about four minutes per side, keeping an eye on it to make sure it doesn't burn. (Cooking time will vary based on the thickness of meat.)

Place green beans and carrots into a large microwave-safe bowl. Add garlic if using. Cover and heat, according to package directions, until steamed.

While meat and vegetables are cooking, mix dill into sour cream, adding salt and pepper to taste. Heat rolls according to package directions.

Serve:

To serve, place 1 cup of beans and carrots on plate, along with one piece of chicken. Drizzle 1 tablespoon of sauce over each piece of chicken and squeeze lemon wedges over vegetables, if desired. Serve with 1 cup skim milk, ½ cup grapes, and a whole-grain roll.

Your serving:

3 oz chicken breast (94 calories, 1 g fat)
½ c green beans (17 calories)
½ c carrots (26 calories)
1 whole-grain roll (80 calories, 1.5 g fat)
1 T light sour cream (20 calories)
1 c skim milk (90 calories)

Total: 375 calories, 2.5 g fat

EASY BLACK BEANS AND RICE (SERVES 4)

2 c canned black beans, drained and rinsed
1½ T taco seasoning (see recipe on page 178)
2 c salsa
4 c baby spinach, washed
1 red bell pepper, chopped
2 c brown rice, cooked according to package directions

Optional: 1 small onion, chopped, and 2 cloves garlic, minced

Preparation:
Spritz a medium skillet with nonstick cooking spray and set over medium heat. Add peppers (and onions if using). Cook about two minutes to allow vegetables to soften, and then add garlic (optional) and taco seasoning. Cook one more minute, then lower heat slightly and add beans and salsa. Simmer for five minutes.

Serve:
To serve, place ½ cup brown rice in a bowl, then top with 1 cup baby spinach. Add 1 cup of the beans and salsa mixture. The heat from the beans will wilt the spinach.
Serve with a cup of soy milk and ½ cup of pineapple.

Your serving:
½ c black beans (114 calories, 0.5 g fat)
½ c salsa (35 calories)
1 c baby spinach (7 calories)
¼ bell pepper (13 calories)
½ c brown rice (108 calories, 1 g fat)
1 c calcium-fortified soy milk (100 calories, 4 g fat)
½ c strawberries (23 calories)

Total: 400 calories, 5.5 g fat

Snacks

Snack time is not an opportunity to forget all the lessons you've learned about eating right and load up on empty calories. Snacks *can* help give you a boost of energy in the afternoon or tide you over until morning. Try to include heart-healthy fats, whole-grain carbs, and protein in your snacks. Snacks are also a great time to work in an extra serving of fruit or vegetables.

Indulging in small treats is an important part of learning to eat right. Treating yourself occasionally can help prevent binges later on. Instead of heading to the vending machine when the 3:00 P.M. munchies set in or a wave of fatigue hits, grab a healthful snack of about 200 calories.

Here are some ideas to get you started. We've included a few sweet snacks, too.

- Fruit and yogurt
- Nuts
- Oatmeal
- Cereal (with more than 3 grams fiber) and milk
- Trail mix with nuts and dried fruit
- Hummus and raw veggies
- Hard-boiled eggs (or egg whites)
- Cottage cheese and fruit
- Half a peanut-butter, turkey, or chicken sandwich on whole-grain bread
- Whole-grain crackers with nut butter or cheese
- Whole-grain fig (or fruit) bars
- Milk (especially chocolate milk)
- Tomato or vegetable juice
- Yogurt smoothie (with added protein powder, if desired)
- Most protein/energy bars

Want something a bit more creative (and specific)? Try the snack ideas below.

- Chop 1 ounce part-skim mozzarella cheese and 6 fresh basil leaves, then mix with 1 cup halved cherry tomatoes. 100 calories, 4.5 grams fat.

- Sprinkle 1 tablespoon Parmesan cheese over 2 cups air-popped popcorn. 85 calories, 1.5 grams fat.

- Top half a medium apple with a 1 ounce slice of low-fat extra-sharp Cheddar cheese. 90 calories, 1 gram fat.

- Wrap 1½ ounces low-sodium turkey deli meat around one small sliced apple. 100 calories, 1 gram fat.

- Top 2 ounces 1% milkfat cottage cheese with one medium peach, sliced. 80 calories, 1 gram fat.

- Mix 2 tablespoons dried cranberries with 2 tablespoons pistachios. 178 calories, 7.4 grams fat.

- Break 1 sheet of graham crackers in two. Place 1 jumbo marshmallow and 1 dark-chocolate kiss atop one half, then top with the second kiss. Microwave a few seconds, until melted and gooey. 110 calories, 1.4 grams fat.

- Spread 1 slice whole-wheat bread with 1 tablespoon natural, low-sodium peanut butter and 1 teaspoon all-fruit spread. 205 calories, 12 grams fat.

- Slice 1 medium banana down the middle and fill with 1 tablespoon cashew butter. Dust with cinnamon. 204 calories, 8.5 grams fat.

- Dunk 2 fig cookies in 1 cup skim milk. 185 calories, 0.5 grams fat.

- Alternate eating 4 dark-chocolate kisses and 1 ounce whole-wheat pretzels. 210 calories, 6.6 grams fat.

- Into ½ cup fat-free Greek yogurt, swirl 1 tablespoon honey. 164 calories, 0 grams fat.

- Mix ½ cup grapes and ½ ounce walnuts. 141 calories, 9 grams fat.

- Nibble on 1 frozen 100% fruit bar. 90 calories, 0 grams fat.

- Top ½ cup fat-free vanilla pudding with ¼ cup strawberries. 145 calories, ½ grams fat.

- Top ½ cup 2% milkfat cottage cheese with ½ cup raspberries. Serve with 8 whole-grain reduced-fat crackers. 176 calories, 4 grams fat.

- Eat ½ cup low-fat chocolate pudding with 1 sheet graham crackers. 119 calories, 3 grams fat.

SAMPLE MEAL PLANS

Using our simple recipes and SparkPeople Mix-and-Match, we've created two sample meal plans to demonstrate how simple and easy eating healthfully can be. These are just examples of how our meal charts can be used to create healthful, efficient meals.

These two days of menus are based on an average 1,500-calorie daily intake and meet the SparkPeople guidelines for proportions of carbohydrates, fats, and proteins. Plus, they prove how easy and delicious it can be to eat several servings of fruits and vegetables throughout the day.

• DAY ONE •

BREAKFAST

Mix:
1 large sliced banana (106 calories)
4 oz low-fat strawberry yogurt (99 calories, 1 g fat)

Sprinkle with:
1 T ground flaxseed (30 calories, 2 g fat)

Split:
1 whole-wheat mini bagel (110 calories, 1 g fat)(144 calories, 2 g fat)

Spread with:
1 t margarine (optional) (34 calories, 4 g fat)

> *Totals: 429 calories • 9 g fat • 82 g carbs • 14 g protein*

LUNCH

Toss:
1 c chopped romaine lettuce (8 calories)
2 c spinach or mixed baby greens (14 calories)

Top with:
3 oz grilled chicken (94 calories, 1 g fat)
½ c shredded or chopped carrots (26 calories)
1 medium tomato, chopped (25 calories)

Drizzle with:
2 T low-fat ranch dressing (80 calories, 4 g fat)

Serve with:
1 whole-grain dinner roll (87 calories, 2 g fat)

> *Totals: 334 calories • 7 g fat • 34 g carbs • 27 g protein*

SNACK 1

Top:
½ c 2% milkfat cottage cheese (81 calories, 2 g fat) with
½ c raspberries (30 calories)

Serve with:
8 whole-grain, reduced-fat crackers (65 calories, 2 g fat)

> *Totals: 176 calories • 4 g fat • 21 g carbs • 6 g protein*

DINNER

Cook:
3 oz 96% lean ground beef (150 calories, 4.5 g fat) in a nonstick skillet with homemade taco seasoning (a pinch each of cumin, chili powder, and paprika) until no longer pink

Add:
½ c fresh salsa* (36 calories) and heat through

Place atop:
1, 6" corn tortilla (57 calories, 1 g fat)

Top with:
¼ c chopped tomatoes (10 calories)
½ c shredded romaine lettuce (4 calories)

Drizzle on:
1 T low-fat sour cream (20 calories, 2 g fat)

Serve alongside:
½ c steamed broccoli (12 calories)
½ c mandarin oranges canned in juice (36 calories)
1 c skim milk (90 calories)

> *Totals: 415 calories • 7.5 g fat • 44 g carbs • 38 g protein*

*Fresh salsa is found in the refrigerated section of the produce department and contains less sodium than jarred varieties. Make your own by chopping 3 large tomatoes, 1 small white onion, 2 cloves garlic, and a handful of fresh cilantro leaves. Season with the juice of half a lime and a pinch of salt.

SNACK 2

Toast:
1 whole-wheat mini-bagel (110 calories, 1 g fat)

Spread with:
2 t natural, low-sodium peanut butter (69 calories, 5 g fat)

> *Totals: 179 calories • 6 g fat • 24 g carbs • 7 g protein*

DAILY TOTALS

*1,533 calories • 33.5 g fat • 205 g carbs • 102 g protein
32 g fiber • 1,996 mg sodium • 3 servings fruit • 6 servings vegetables*

• DAY TWO •

BREAKFAST

Toast:
1 whole-grain English muffin (120 calories, 1 g fat)

Top with:
1 egg, poached or boiled (74 calories, 5 g fat)
2 slices turkey bacon cooked according to package directions (34 calories, 3 g fat)
1 oz low-fat Cheddar cheese (50 calories, 2 g fat)

Serve with:
½ large orange (44 calories)
1 c skim milk (90 calories, 0 g fat)

Totals: 412 calories • 11 g fat • 47 g carbs • 31 g protein

LUNCH

Begin with:
1 t Dijon mustard (5 calories) spread on
2 slices whole-grain bread (130 calories, 2 g fat)

Assemble sandwich with:
3 oz low-sodium, lean ham (90 calories, 1 g fat)
1 slice low-fat Swiss cheese (45 calories, 3 g fat)
1 large leaf romaine lettuce (2 calories)
3 tomato slices (13 calories)

Serve with:
½ c grapes (48 calories)
½ c baby carrots (26 calories)

Totals: 359 calories • 6 g fat • 50 g carbs • 21 g protein

SNACK 1

Eat:
½ c low-fat chocolate pudding (60 calories, 2 g fat)
1 sheet graham crackers (59 calories, 1 g fat)

Totals: 119 calories • 3 g fat • 24 g carbs • 3 g protein

DINNER

Top:
3 oz chicken breast (94 calories, 1 g fat) with homemade barbecue sauce* (52 calories) and grill or bake at 400 degrees Fahrenheit until chicken is no longer pink and juices run clear

Serve with:
1 c skim milk (90 calories, 0 g fat)
½ c frozen peas (55 calories)
½ c green beans (17 calories)
½ c baked sweet potato (70 calories)
½ c cantaloupe (32 calories)

Totals: 410 calories • 1 g fat • 62 g carbs • 36 g protein

*To make sauce: Mince one clove of garlic, then mix with 1 t brown sugar, ½ T cider vinegar, and 2 T no-salt-added tomato paste. Season to taste and spread on chicken before cooking.

SNACK 2

Spread:
1 slice whole-wheat bread (86 calories, 3 g fat) with
1 T natural, low-sodium peanut butter (105 calories, 9 g fat) and
1 t all-fruit spread (14 calories)

Totals: 205 calories • 12 g fat • 23 g carbs • 6 g protein

DAILY TOTALS

1,505 calories • 33 g fat • 206 g carbs • 97 g protein
2,200 mg sodium • 27 g fiber • 3 servings fruit • 4 servings vegetables

SUPERFOODS

Another great way to make small changes that can make a big difference to your health is to rev up the nutritional punch of your meals and snacks by adding "superfoods."

These foods power your brain and efficiently fuel your body. Superfoods may also fight infection, enhance your immune system, and protect against diseases such as osteoporosis, heart disease, certain cancers, diabetes, and respiratory infections.

While our list of superfoods may be longer than most, it shows that great things do come in small packages. These foods are not only healthy, but they're also affordable, familiar, and readily available at regular grocery stores and farmers markets. With so many choices, you'll discover just how easy it is to eat super-healthy every day . . . even on a tight budget.

Some of these foods might not be right for your tastes, preferences, or health goals. Remember, no single food can provide everything you need to be healthy. That's why it's important to choose a variety of superfoods from each category to meet your daily nutrition needs. One way some members do this is by hanging this list on the refrigerator. Every week when they make a shopping list, they pick out a few "new" superfoods that they don't usually buy and add them to the list.

To find recipes that use these superfoods, go to SparkRecipes.com and enter the name of any superfood into the keyword search.

Vegetables

Asparagus	Cauliflower	Mustard greens	Spinach
Avocados	Collard greens	Onions	Summer squash
Beets	Crimini mushrooms	Peas	Sweet potatoes
Bell peppers	Cucumbers	Portobello mushrooms	Swiss chard
Broccoli	Eggplant	Potatoes	Tomatoes
Brussels Sprouts	Garlic	Rainbow chard	Turnip greens
Cabbage	Green beans	Romaine lettuce	Winter squash
Carrots	Kale	Shiitake mushrooms	Yams

Fruits

Apples	Cherries	Lemons	Pineapple
Apricots	Cranberries	Limes	Plums
Bananas	Figs	Nectarines	Prunes
Black olives	Grapefruit	Oranges	Raisins
Blackberries	Grapes	Papaya	Raspberries
Blueberries	Honeydew melon	Peaches	Strawberries
Cantaloupe	Kiwifruit	Pears	Watermelon

Grains

Amaranth	Bulgur	Quinoa	Whole-grain bread
Arborio rice	Corn	Rye	Whole-grain cereal
Barley	Jasmine rice	Spelt	Whole-grain pasta
Brown rice	Millet	Triticale	Wild rice
Buckwheat	Oats	Wheat berries	

Calcium-Rich Foods

Almond milk	Cottage cheese (low-fat)	Orange juice with calcium	Soy milk
Cheese (low-fat)	Milk (skim or 1%)	Rice milk	Yogurt with active cultures (low-fat)

Protein

Almonds	Flaxseed	Peanut butter (natural)	Sunflower seeds
Beef (lean)	Hemp seeds	Peanuts	Tahini
Black beans	Hummus	Pinto beans	Tempeh
Cashews	Kidney beans	Pork (lean)	Tofu
Chicken (skinless)	Lima beans	Pumpkin seeds	Tuna (canned or fresh)
Chickpeas (garbanzo beans)	Lentils	Salmon (canned or fresh)	Turkey (skinless)
Egg whites	Miso	Seafood (unbreaded)	Veggie burgers
Eggs	Navy beans	Sesame seeds	Walnuts
Fish (unbreaded)	Nuts	Soybeans	Wild game (skinless)

Miscellaneous

Canola oil	Dark chocolate	Green tea	Olive oil

THE SPARK
10-MINUTE WORKOUTS

As we said earlier, we love 10-minute workouts. They're easy to fit in no matter how busy you are, they are great for people just starting an exercise program, and if you already exercise, they can make a big difference in how consistently you exercise. You can almost always use a 10-minute workout as a fallback when you don't have time for more. That way, you won't fall off the workout wagon altogether when you get busy, and you'll keep your body moving and your momentum going.

In this section, SparkPeople's Coach Nicole has created five 10-minute workout options that you can do at home; four of them don't even require any equipment at all, so they are especially accessible to anyone. There are two strength-training workouts and three cardio options. Remember, we recommend that you do at least two strength-training workouts per week on nonconsecutive days. Both of the strength-training workouts here are full-body workouts, so you can do one of these twice a week or do a different one each time. We also recommend that you do some kind of cardio workout at least three and preferably four times per week. For cardio, feel free to do anything you like—walk, run, elliptical trainer, Stairmaster—or use one of Coach Nicole's 10-minute cardio routines below. We've also added a fun option here that lets you create your own cardio workout using basic aerobic moves that you can mix and match!

As with any program, check with your doctor before you begin if you haven't exercised in a while or if you have any health problems.

STRENGTH-TRAINING WORKOUTS

Get a jump on your strength training with these 10-minute routines that you can do at home! We designed these workouts to work out each of the important muscle groups for a full-body workout in 10 minutes or less. We selected exercises that specifically work more than one muscle group at once so that you get maximum results in a shorter time. We recommend you do one set to fit your workout into the 10-minute time frame, but if you have time, or once you work up to it, feel free to do two sets of each exercise.

Be sure to warm up before your workout, perform exercises in the order listed (do one set of ten repetitions unless otherwise noted), and stretch when you're finished. For stretching ideas, visit SparkPeople.com.

10-Minute Equipment-Free Workout

Wide-Leg Squat, Pop & Drop

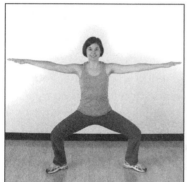 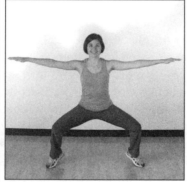 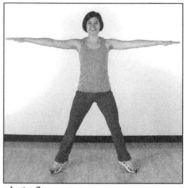

photo 1   photo 2   photo 3

Starting position: Stand tall with feet more than hip width apart, toes turned out, abs engaged, and arms extended at shoulder level (not pictured).

Action: Inhale and bend your knees to lower straight down into a squat (photo 1). From there, "pop" your heels up off the ground (photo 2). Exhale, keeping heels lifted, and straighten your legs to stand tall (photo 3). Once legs are straight, "drop" your heels back down to the floor to complete one rep and return to the starting position. Repeat.

Special instructions: Keep your back straight, chest lifted, glutes tucked under, knees and toes pointed in the same direction, and knees behind your toes when squatting. To aid your balance when on the balls of your feet, fix your gaze on a focal point in front of you.

Bridges

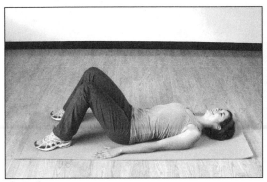
photo 1

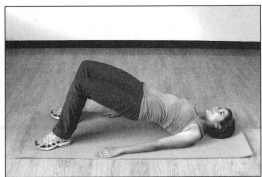
photo 2

Starting position: Lie on your back with abs engaged, arms on the floor at your sides, feet flat, knees bent, and legs hip width apart (photo 1).

Action: Exhale and bridge your hips up toward the ceiling, squeezing your glutes and hamstrings at the top (photo 2). Inhale and lower back down to the starting position to complete one rep. Repeat.

Special instructions: Push your weight into your heels. Do not put any pressure on your head or neck. Keep your abs engaged to protect your lower back.

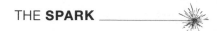
Side Push-ups

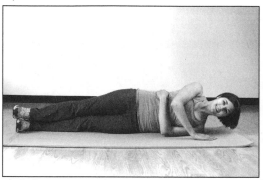
photo 1

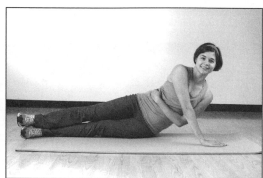
photo 2

Starting position: Lie on your right side with abs engaged, legs straight and stacked. Place your top (left) hand flat on the floor in front of your shoulder, elbow bent, and your bottom (right) arm wrapped around your waist (photo 1).

Action: Exhale and push your body up, straightening your top (left) arm and laterally flexing your spine as if bringing your top shoulder toward your hip (photo 2). Inhale and slowly bend your elbow to return to the starting position to complete one rep. Repeat; switch sides.

Special instructions: Don't let your legs lift off the floor. Keep your abs engaged and your head and neck neutral. Relax your shoulders away from your ears.

Plank

Starting position: Lie facedown on the mat with abs engaged. Clasp your hands and place your elbows under your shoulders with your forearms flat, toes curled under, and legs together (not pictured). Lift your weight off the mat, balancing on your elbows, forearms, and toes, while maintaining a straight line from your shoulders to your feet (photo 1). Pull your belly away from the floor underneath you.

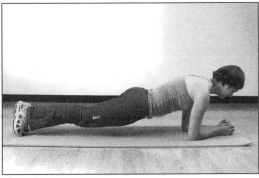

photo 1

Action: Breathe naturally and hold the plank position for 15 seconds, gradually building up your endurance over time until you can hold for one minute.

Special instructions: Keep your abs engaged. Balance your weight evenly between your elbows/forearms and your feet. Keep your shoulders pulled back. Make sure your hips do not droop toward the floor.

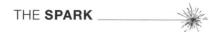

Push-ups

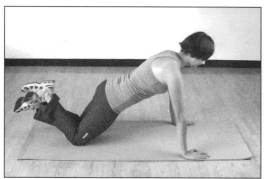
photo 1

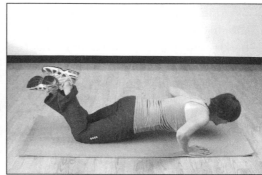
photo 2

Starting position: Kneel on your mat and place your hands on the floor, directly under your shoulders. Engage your abs and lower your hips toward the floor until your body is in a straight line from your shoulders to your knees (photo 1).

Action: Inhale and bend your elbows to lower your body toward the floor (photo 2). Exhale to push back up to the starting position to complete one rep. Repeat.

Special instructions: Lower your body only as far as you can while maintaining a straight line from the shoulders to the knees. If strong enough, perform push-ups on your toes instead of your knees.

T-Arm Back Extensions

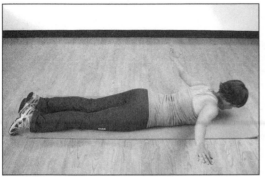 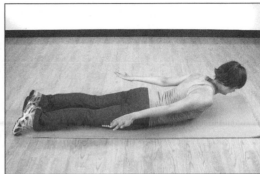

photo 1   photo 2

Starting position: Lie flat on your stomach, legs extended on the mat behind you, arms extended at your sides like a T, head and neck in a neutral position, and arms hovering above the floor with your shoulders pulled back (photo 1).

Action: Exhale, pulling your abs in tight and engaging your lower back, to lift your chest away from the floor as you sweep your arms toward your hips and squeeze your shoulder blades together (photo 2). Inhale and return to the starting position to complete one rep. Repeat.

Special instructions: Keep your abs engaged. Keep your neck neutral and in line with your spine. Lift your chest only as high as you can without hurting your lower back. Don't let your shoulders round forward or touch the floor—not even in the starting position.

10-Minute Strength-Training Workout with Dumbbells

Dumbbell Squat with Overhead Press

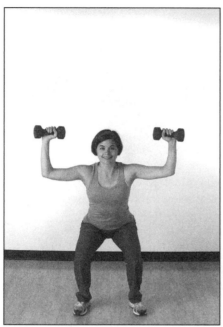 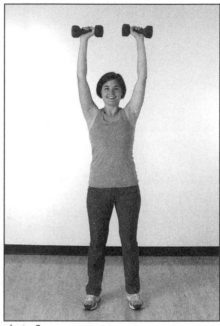

photo 1   photo 2

Starting position: Stand with your feet hip width apart, back straight, toes pointing forward, abs engaged, one weight in each hand, elbows bent and weights held above your shoulders, palms facing forward. Bend your knees and hips, lowering into a squat position as if sitting back into a chair behind you (photo 1).

Action: Exhale and straighten your knees to push up out of your squat as you push your weights overhead in line with your shoulders (photo 2). Inhale to slowly squat back down and return the weights to the starting position to complete one rep. Repeat.

Special instructions: Keep your chest lifted and try to minimize any forward leaning. Push your weight back into your heels and don't let your knees come farther forward than your toes.

Right-Leg Lunge with Biceps Curls

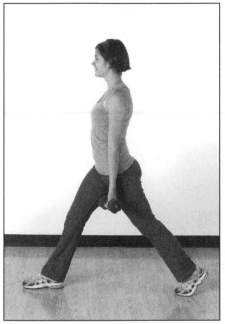 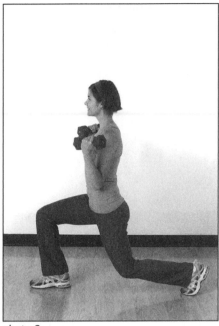

photo 1   photo 2

Starting position: Stand tall with your right leg staggered in front of your left leg, abs engaged, back straight, toes pointing forward, weights in each hand, elbows at your sides and palms facing up (photo 1).

Action: Exhale and bend both knees to lunge straight down as you curl the weights up toward your shoulders (photo 2). Inhale to straighten the legs, lower the weights, and return to the starting position to complete one rep. Repeat for ten reps, but do not switch sides—move on to the next exercise instead.

Special instructions: When lunging, keep your back straight and avoid leaning forward. Make sure your front knee does not move forward of your toes. Lunge down only as far as you can with good form.

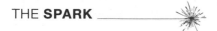

Left-Leg Lunge with Shoulder Raises

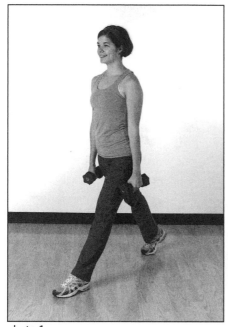

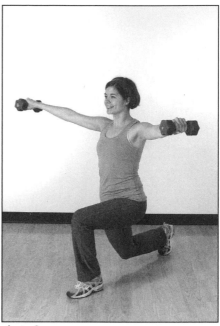

photo 1

photo 2

Starting position: Stand tall with your left leg staggered in front of your right leg, abs engaged, back straight, toes pointing forward, weights in each hand, arms at your sides, and palms facing in (photo 1).

Action: Exhale and bend both knees to lunge straight down as you raise your arms from your sides up to shoulder height (photo 2). Inhale to straighten your legs, lower the weights, and return to the starting position to complete one rep. Repeat for ten reps, but do not switch sides.

Special instructions: See previous exercise.

Rows with Triceps Extensions

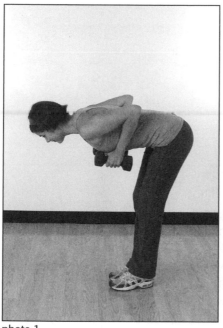 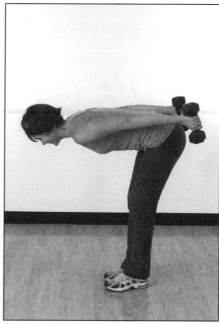

photo 1   photo 2

Starting position: Holding one weight in each hand, stand tall with feet together, abs engaged, knees slightly bent, and back straight. Pull your belly in tight and bend over from the waist until your back is flat and parallel to the floor and your arms are hanging straight down below your shoulders, palms facing in.

Action: Exhale and slowly row the weights up toward your chest, keeping your arms close to your sides, bending your elbows, and squeezing your shoulder blades together (photo 1). Inhale and straighten your elbows, lifting the weights back and up toward the ceiling behind you (photo 2). Exhale to bend the elbows again (photo 1), then inhale to lower the weights back down to the starting position to complete one rep. Repeat.

Special instructions: Always keep your abs engaged to help protect your lower back in this position. Keep your head and neck in line with the spine. If this position bothers your lower back or you cannot maintain a flat back, perform this exercise while seated on a ball or chair (bent over your thighs) instead of standing.

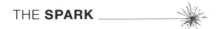

Bridges with Chest Press

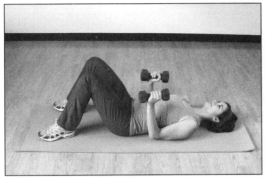

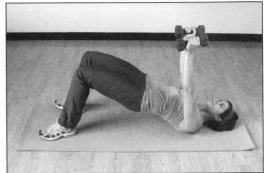

photo 1   photo 2

Starting position: Lie on your back with abs engaged, feet flat, knees bent, weights in each hand, elbows bent, and palms facing in (photo 1).

Action: Exhale and bridge your hips up toward the ceiling, squeezing your glutes and hamstrings at the top, and push your weights up toward the ceiling, straightening your arms (photo 2). Inhale and lower back down to the starting position to complete one rep. Repeat.

Special instructions: Push your weight into your heels. Do not put any pressure on your head or neck. Always keep your abs engaged to protect your lower back.

Bicycle Crunches

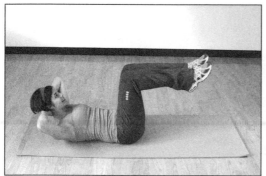
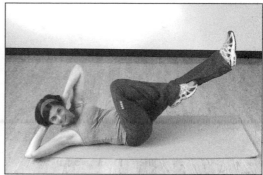

photo 1   photo 2

Starting position: Lie on your back with your abs engaged, knees bent and in line with the hips, shins parallel to the floor, lower back flat on the floor, and hands behind your head for light support. Engage your abs to crunch up, lifting your head, neck, and shoulder blades off the mat (photo 1).

Action: Exhale, twisting from the waist to bring your left elbow toward your right knee as your left leg extends away from the body (photo 2). Inhale and return to the starting position (photo 1). Switch sides (exhale to bring your right elbow toward your left knee as your right leg extends) to complete one rep. Repeat.

Special instructions: Keep your abs engaged and your lower back flat. Do not use your arms or hands to help you lift your head, neck, and shoulders—use them only to support the neck.

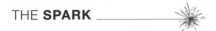

Back Extensions

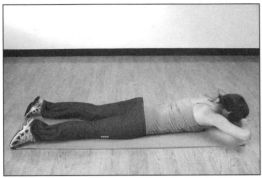
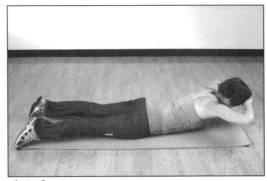

photo 1   photo 2

Starting position: Lie face down on your mat, legs extended in line with your hips, abs engaged, elbows bent, arms hovering above the floor, and hands supporting your fore-head (photo 1). Pull your shoulders back, away from the mat.

Action: Exhale, engaging your lower back muscles as you lift your chest away from the floor, head resting on your hands (photo 2). Inhale to slowly lower to the starting position to complete one rep. Repeat.

Special instructions: Keep your abs engaged. Lift your chest only as high as you can without feeling pain in your lower back. Don't let your shoulders round forward or touch the floor—not even in the starting position.

CARDIO WORKOUTS

You can get your cardio in whatever way you like best. We always recommend that people try different things and find what they like. Some people love a gym workout with machines and the active environment, where they're surrounded by others working out. Others like the fresh air and peace they get with a walk through a park. Some like the convenience and privacy of working out at home. Many like to mix it up and try different things to stay motivated. Here, we provide a unique at-home option that you can use whenever you want, for as long as you want.

Mix-and-Match Cardio Options: Create Your Own Workouts!

Cardio doesn't have to be complicated. When you use SparkPeople's Mix-and-Match Cardio options, it's as if you have a fitness trainer creating new workouts for you, right in your own home. All of these exercises, when done long enough, can elevate your heart rate to an aerobic level. While all of these moves vary in intensity and complexity, you're sure to find some moves that work for you. Play your favorite songs, keep up with the beat of the music, and don't forget—it should be fun!

Here's how to create your own Mix-and-Match workouts:

- Always warm up for a few minutes with light exercise before you start and cool down for a few minutes when you're finished. Don't forget to stretch after you work out either. (You'll find plenty of stretching ideas at SparkPeople.com.)

- 10-minute workouts are a great way to start, but you can use these ideas to work out for any length of time that suits your schedule and fitness level.

- Remember to work at your own level. To make any move easier, go slower, minimize your arm movement (or omit it completely), or make your range of motion smaller. To make any exercise more challenging, increase your speed and/or range of motion.

- Once you start your workout, try to stay moving—go from one move to the next without rest. If you get tired, never stop abruptly without cooling down first. If you need to rest or catch your breath, do a slow march in place as long as you need to.

15 Mix-and-Match Moves

Below, you'll find 15 simple cardio moves you can use to create your own cardio workouts at home—no equipment necessary! For workout ideas, refer to the three sample workouts that Coach Nicole created (below), or create your own—picking your five favorite moves, for example, and then doing each for two minutes at a time to complete a ten-minute session. It's that easy! You control the pace, speed, and range of movement to suit your own fitness level.

1. *Marching.* Stand tall (abs in, back straight, shoulders down, and elbows bent) and march in place, pumping your arms at your sides.

2. *High knee grab.* Stand tall (abs in, back straight, shoulders down, and elbows bent). Step on your right foot and reach your arms overhead. Then lift your left foot off the ground, driving your knee toward the ceiling and pulling your arms down, elbows toward your knee. When you place your left foot down, reach overhead again, then pull your arms down and lift your right knee. Repeat.

3. *Jumping jacks.* A classic cardio move! Hop out to make the shape of an X with your arms and legs and then hop back in (legs together and arms down). Repeat.

4. *Front jabs.* Punch one arm straight out in front of your shoulder and then pull it back in, keeping the other arm up, elbow bent, as if in "defense." Repeat. (Note that you can jab with one arm at a time or alternate arms.)

5. *Jogging in place.* Stand tall (abs in, back straight, shoulders down, and elbows bent) and jog in place, pumping your arms at your sides and bringing your heels up behind you. Repeat.

6. *High-knee jogging in place.* Stand tall (abs in, back straight, shoulders down, and elbows bent) and jog in place, pumping your arms at your sides and bringing your knees up in front of you. Repeat.

7. *Squat thrusts.* Stand tall (abs in, back straight, shoulders down). Squat deeply, bending your knees and hips until your hands touch the floor in front of you. Jump back into a plank position (hands under your shoulders, legs straight behind you, abs in tight). Jump back in to your low squat. Stand back up to the starting position. Repeat.

8. *Mountain climbers.* Squat down to the floor and jump out to a plank position (hands under your shoulders, legs straight behind you, abs in tight). Hold that position as you "jog" in place, bringing one knee at a time toward your chest, alternating feet. Repeat.

9. *Squat and reach.* Stand tall (abs in, back straight, shoulders down) with feet wider than hip width apart. Squat straight down, reaching your fingertips toward the floor, then push back up, reaching your arms straight up overhead. Repeat.

10. *Front kicks.* Stand tall (abs in, back straight, shoulders down) with feet hip width apart, elbows bent, arms up in defense. To kick, lift your knee, extend your leg (foot flexed), then bend your knee again and lower your foot to the floor to complete one rep. Repeat. (Note that you can kick with a single leg at a time or alternate legs.)

11. *Speed skating.* Stand tall (abs in, back straight, shoulders down, and elbows bent) with feet hip width apart. Hop laterally to the right to land softly on your right foot, then let your left toes tap the floor behind your right leg. Then hop laterally to the left to land softly on your left foot, then let your right toes tap the floor behind your left leg. Repeat.

12. *Step-touch.* Stand tall (abs in, back straight, shoulders down, hands on hips). Move side to side with the following foot pattern: right step (to the side), left touch (next to the right foot), left step (to the side), right touch (next to the left foot). Repeat side to side. To make it easier, take smaller steps and/or don't move your arms.

13. *Grapevines.* Stand tall (abs in, back straight, shoulders down, hands on hips). Step to the right, following this foot pattern: right step (to the side), left step (behind right foot), right step (to the side), left touch (next to the right foot). Repeat in the opposite direction: left step (to the side), right step (behind the left foot), left step (to the side), right touch (next to the right foot). Repeat side to side.

14. *V-steps.* Stand tall (abs in, back straight, shoulders down, hands on hips, feet together). Picture a V on the floor with your feet standing on the bottom point. Move forward and back with the following foot pattern: right step (forward) toward the right point of the V, left step (forward) toward the left point of the V, right step (back) to the bottom point of the V, and left step (back) to the bottom point of the V. Repeat.

15. *Faux jumping rope.* Stand tall (abs in, back straight, shoulders down, elbows bent, hands wide, feet together). Circle your wrists and imagine you are turning a jump rope. Hop off the floor to clear your rope. Repeat.

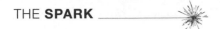

Sample 10-Minute Mix-and-Match Cardio Workouts

All of these workouts show how you can use the moves above to create a cardio workout that lasts for ten minutes. For a longer workout, do each move longer than the suggested time or repeat all or part of the series.

Workout 1

1. Warm up
2. Marching (2 minutes)
3. Step-touch (1 minute)
4. Grapevines (1 minute)
5. Jogging in place (1 minute)
6. Faux jumping rope (1 minute)
7. Speed skating (1 minute)
8. Squat and reach (1 minute)
9. High-knee jogging in place (2 minutes)
10. Cool down and stretch

Workout 2

1. Warm up
2. Squat and reach (1 minute)
3. Front jabs, alternating arms (1 minute)
4. Front kicks, alternating legs (1 minute)
5. Faux jumping rope (2 minutes)
6. Squat thrusts (1 minute)
7. Step-touch (1 minute)
8. Jumping jacks (2 minutes)
9. Jogging in place (1 minute)
10. Cool down and stretch.

Workout 3

1. Warm up
2. Grapevines (1 minute)
3. V-steps (1 minute)

4. High knee grabs (2 minutes)
5. Mountain climbers (1 minute)
6. High-knee jogging in place (1 minute)
7. Front kicks (1 minute)
8. Speed skating (2 minutes)
9. Faux jumping rope (1 minute)
10. Cool down and stretch.

HEALTHY LIFESTYLE PLEDGE

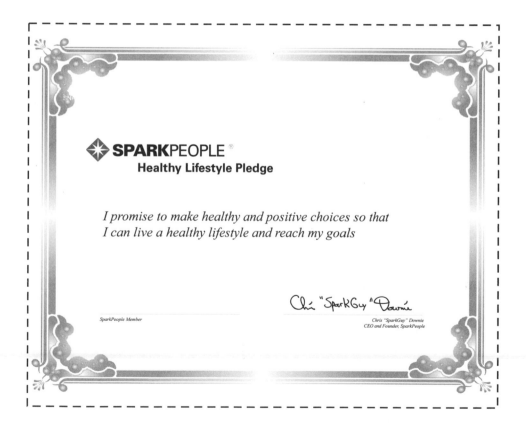

SPARKPEOPLE ®
Healthy Lifestyle Pledge

*I promise to make healthy and positive choices so that
I can live a healthy lifestyle and reach my goals*

SparkPeople Member

Chris "SparkGuy" Downie
CEO and Founder, SparkPeople

SPARKPOINTS

Competition is a great way to stay motivated! Almost half of our successful members use some kind of competitive activity as a motivational tool, and many of them do so by keeping track of SparkPoints on SparkPeople.com. We designed SparkPoints to encourage members to take steps that are proven to help them reach their goals—tasks and activities ranging from working out to tracking food to supporting others in the online community. Each healthy action they take earns them points.

SparkPoints can make your journey through this book more exciting, too. See below to learn how you can earn SparkPoints for reading each chapter and completing the Action Steps—and what rewards await you when you do!

PRIZES

We will have a drawing at least every three months. Anyone who earns at least 900 SparkPoints from reading the book and completing the Action Steps will be eligible for the prizes. One person per month will win this prize package:

- $100 gift certificate to the SparkPeople store
- SparkGuy Award autographed by me
- Congratulatory phone call from me

To enter your points online, simply go to SparkPeople.com/TheSpark.

Here's a rundown of the SparkPoints you can earn just from reading *The Spark:*

Chapter	Points
1	50
2	50
3	50
4	50
5	50
6	50
7	50
8	50
9	50
Total Reading Points	450

And here's how you can earn points for taking each healthy step in the book. Note: Give yourself 25 points for completing part of the goals for a week. If you do the total goals for a week in the future, you can go back and credit yourself with the full 50 points for that week.

Book Activity	Points
Setting Goals (Chapter 2)	75
Chapter 6 Action Steps	75
Chapter 7 Action Steps	75
Chapter 8 Action Steps	75
Chapter 9 Action Steps	75
Total Book Activity Points	375

Finally, here are some other ways to earn SparkPoints:

Other Activity	Points
Join SparkPeople.com	50
Join The Spark SparkTeam	25
Get others to read *The Spark* (25 points per person, up to 100 points total)	100
Earn SparkPoints for using SparkPeople.com (these are tracked automatically by the Website—you can earn over 100 points per day for using the site!)	See Website
Total Other Activity Points	175+

That's a total of 1,000+ SparkPoints you can earn from using this book and joining our community of SparkPeople!

SPARKPEOPLE SECRETS OF SUCCESS MEMBER SURVEY RESULTS

For the first time ever, we have done a member survey, drawing from among our millions of members, and analyzed its results to quantify the specific tools, behaviors, attitudes, and mindsets that make our most successful members so successful. And we're sharing them with you so that we can help you increase your odds of making a healthy lifestyle change. You've heard a lot about our findings in the chapters you've already read. Here's the full story of how we conducted the survey and what we learned.

METHODOLOGY

We sent a 64-question survey via e-mail to a random sample of our active members. We received over 5,500 completed responses. From there, we segmented out different groups to see what we could learn. We looked at "100-pound losers," those who had lost at least 100 pounds (and many of whom had lost much more); this group included both members who had already reached their goals and those still working toward their goals. We examined "Successfully met goal" members, those who had reached their weight loss goals. And we looked at the "stuck," members who had not met their goals and reported that they were not on track to reach them. When we refer to "successful members" here and throughout the book, we often mean both those who have already met their final goals plus those who have lost 100 pounds *and* say they are on track to lose the rest.

When we refer to "dieters," we mean people who are less likely to make a healthy lifestyle change—these people are following plans typically associated with "yo-yo dieting," as opposed to those members who are making a real change in the way they live ("healthy

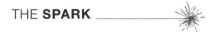

lifestyle members") and they actually labeled their own weight loss efforts as "dieting" versus "pursuing a healthy lifestyle."

What did we learn? We'll give you some of the highlights here that will show you:

- How our members have lost between 2 and 200 pounds—or more!

- How so many of our members went from being winded after walking to the mailbox to running in their first marathons

- How the majority of respondents report significantly higher levels of confidence, improved sex lives, greater health and fitness levels, the achievement of goals beyond their weight-loss goals, improved relationships, and even significantly improved measures of happiness

While a segment of members used most of the SparkPeople secrets of success most of the time, (with great success), the majority of our successful members varied which strategies they used at a particular time—depending on their goals and what's going on in their lives. One of the keys is to use a combination of strategies from the different cornerstones together for the best effect.

SECRETS OF SUCCESS

Goal-Setting Secrets of Success

- *Be a "goal-getter."* Of our successful members, 96 percent were actively working toward one or more goals. They all either had or had met weight loss goals, but they also had active fitness goals (81.5 percent), health-related goals (49 percent), and other life goals like financial, career, relationship, creative pursuits, and many more.

- *Start small to achieve big results.* Almost 80 percent of successful members started with small steps, and once they built a firm foundation, they went from there. Dieters were more likely to start with big goals and go all out trying to lose weight fast.

- *Make a plan.* Of those who met their goals, a full 74 percent planned their meals and workouts in advance, and over 78 percent of 100-pound losers did! And, when compared to those who had not met their goals or were "stuck," successful members planned their workouts more than twice as often.

Nutrition Secrets of Success

- *Stop dieting.* Fully 90 percent of all members said they were following a healthy lifestyle, as opposed to dieting. People on a diet actually lost less weight! There were big differences in how dieters thought. They were twice as likely to think of exercise as a chore, more likely to "beat themselves up," more likely to cut out food groups and deprive themselves, and more likely to say that they "don't feel good about themselves." They got less sleep on average between five and seven hours, versus seven to eight hours in the healthy lifestyle group. Dieters also reported lower levels of happiness.

- *Eat breakfast.* Almost all successful SparkPeople, and all 100-pound losers, either ate a substantial breakfast (66 percent) or ate some breakfast (25.5 percent) every day—so over 90 percent are at least some breakfast every day. Less than 1 percent of the most successful members skipped it altogether.

- *Eat more fruits and veggies.* Across all successful segments, whether it be 100-pound losers or those who had met their weight-loss goals in general, the number-one nutritional strategy was to eat more fruits and vegetables. Of those who met their goals and reached their ideal weight, 90 percent now eat more fruits and veggies.

- *Get cooking.* Cooking healthy meals for yourself is the number-two nutrition strategy of successful members; 77 percent of them used this strategy to meet their goals.

- *Drink water!* Of successful members, 74.5 percent drank eight or more cups of water per day. Only around 50 percent of dieters got enough water.

- *Track your food.* Of those successful, about half tracked their food every day, and most tracked their food sometimes, while only 17 percent of those who said they were not reaching their goal or were stuck tracked their food. While many members no longer track food after reaching their goals—or track just periodically—if you're stuck, sometimes the simplest and most effective thing to do is just start by tracking your food for one day.

- *Follow the 80/20 rule.* Of successful members, 96 percent ate a healthy diet most of the time (between 80 percent and 100 percent) The majority

(70 percent) didn't cut out "bad foods." These members understand that adopting a healthy lifestyle for life is not about perfection. It makes sense, then, that successful members say that when they have a "bad food day," they "don't worry about it because I eat healthy and exercise most of the time" (over 61 percent).

- *Know how much you're eating.* Members were often surprised by how much they had been eating once they began to use the nutrition tracker. And they were often confused by portion sizes at first. To solve this problem, 65 percent of all successful members measured their portions before they ate.

Exercise Secrets of Success

- *Move it to lose it.* Okay, the idea of exercising to lose weight and increase your fitness level is not news. But these survey statistics make a powerful case for it. Of those who reached their goals, 90 percent exercised regularly, and they worked out on average four to six times a week. Only 56 percent of those not meeting their goals exercised, and those who did were more likely to exercise three times a week or less.

- *Don't give up.* Don't like to exercise? Take heart. Of those people who met their goals, only half of them actually liked exercise before they started SparkPeople, but a full 75 percent like it now! (And a full 96 percent either like it, love it, or at least love how it makes them feel when they're done.)

- *Sneak in more exercise.* Sixty-five percent of members added more activity to their day by "sneaking" it in: pacing while on the phone, lifting weights in front of the TV, doing jumping jacks in between conference calls, taking the stairs, Not only does this keep your metabolism going, it also wakes you up when your energy is waning and helps keep your body in motion!

- *Go for strength.* Successful members were twice as likely to do regular strength training. Aside from helping build and maintain a strong and healthy body, these members also know that with more muscle, their bodies will regularly burn more calories, even when they're sleeping.

Motivation Secrets of Success

- *Give yourself a pep talk.* When successful members were asked if they used motivational techniques, they reported their number-one motivational strategy as "I give myself positive self-talk." This technique is hard for some to get used to, but it really works.

- *Your friends can make you thin.* Surround yourself with positive and healthy influences. Successful members had more "healthy friends"—those who supported their healthy lifestyle either by encouraging them or participating with them.

- *Mix it up to keep it up.* Successful members exercised at home, outside, in the gym, with home equipment or home DVDs, and/or with workout groups or buddies, varying their routines and keeping it fun so that they were more likely to keep going.

- *Don't look back.* Of all successful members, 84 percent said that if they hit a setback in their pursuit of weight-loss or fitness goals, they just acknowledged the bump and quickly moved on to get right back on track. Literally zero percent of successful members said that setbacks derailed their efforts.

- *Tap into the power of positive people.* SparkPeople members don't just consider other people a nice part of their community; instead they tap into the power of positive people and use that as a weight-loss tool. Of successful members, 60 percent connected with positive people who they knew would help them stay positive, and 58.6 percent proactively read other people's success stories on SparkPeople.com. Among 100-pound losers, the numbers were even higher—72 percent of those people proactively connected with positive people who they knew would keep them positive, and 71 percent read inspiring stories of other successful SparkPeople.

- *Make it fun.* Successful members proactively took steps to keep exercise fun, including trying new and different things (64.3 percent), doing outdoor activities (67 percent), listening to fun music (62 percent), and purposefully adding variety to their workout plans (58.5 percent). Other things that kept it fun were doing competitive activities (races, charity walks) and taking active vacations.

Secrets of 100-Pound Losers

While many people have come to SparkPeople over the years to lose 5 or 10 or 25 pounds, or to work toward fitness goals independent of weight loss, we also have many members whose weight-loss goals are much larger. As part of our survey analysis, we took at look at those who had successfully lost over 100 pounds, to see if they did anything differently. Many of these people still had additional weight to lose to reach their ultimate goals, but the majority of them were on track to reach those goals. Many others had met their weight-loss goals, losing 100 or 150 pounds or more, and are now at their ideal weight.

While most of their behaviors and attitudes were very similar to those of the larger group of people who had successfully met their weight-loss goals, a few things stood out:

- *More consistent food tracking.* People who lost 100 pounds or more tracked their food at a higher rate and with even more consistency than the rest of the successful members.

- *Water, water everywhere.* They were more likely to drink even more than eight glasses of water per day.

- *Moving more.* They tended to do slightly more cardio and were more likely to strength train more than three days per week.

- *Learning to love it.* Of 100-pound losers, 66 percent did not like exercise before SparkPeople, but after being on the program, they reported a complete flip-flop—now fully 66 percent do like exercise. (This shows the power of reaching the exercise tipping point!)

- *More healthy friends.* A full 22.8 percent of 100-pound losers reported having the highest number of healthy friends in our survey—20 or more—versus only 2 percent of those who said they were stuck. Similarly, 100-pound losers connected more often with positive people who helped them stay motivated (73 percent, versus 59.8 percent of other successful members). By comparison, only 36 percent of those who said they were "stuck" connected with positive people.

How have these 100-pound losers' lives changed as a result? They:

- Feel more confident than before (41.6 percent)
- Report that their sex lives have improved (60 percent)
- Feel like "they can do anything they put their mind to" (32.8 percent)

Of members who had lost 100 pounds or more—even though more than half still had weight to lose—only 3.6 percent said they "don't feel good about themselves." How many of those who were not meeting their goals said they did not feel good about themselves? A whopping 41.6 percent.

TRACKER PAGES

SPARKPEOPLE.com Daily Tracker   DATE: _____   WEIGHT: _____

Nutrition Tracker
FOOD AND DRINK

Breakfast

Daily Goals!

TIME: _____

	Amount:	Calories:	Fat Grams:	Protein Grams:	Carbs Grams:
BREAKFAST TOTALS:					

COMMENTS:

___ Calories

___ Fat

___ Protein

___ Carbohydrates

DAILY SERVING INTAKE

#Fruit Servings

#Vegetable Servings

Cups of Water

Lunch

TIME: _____

	Amount:	Calories:	Fat Grams:	Protein Grams:	Carbs Grams:
LUNCH TOTALS:					

COMMENTS:

Dinner

TIME: _____

	Amount:	Calories:	Fat Grams:	Protein Grams:	Carbs Grams:
DINNER TOTALS:					

COMMENTS:

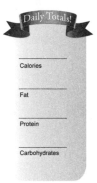

Nutrition Tracker
FOOD AND DRINK

Snacks

	Time:	Amount:	Calories:	Fat Grams:	Protein Grams:	Carbs Grams:
SNACK TOTALS:						
COMMENTS:						

Daily Totals!

Calories

Fat

Protein

Carbohydrates

Exercise and Fitness Tracker
DAILY PHYSICAL ACTIVITIES

Activity / Exercise:	Reps / Sets:	Weight / Level:	Time:	Calories Burned:
TOTAL TIME / TOTAL CALORIES BURNED:				
COMMENTS:				

Goal and Motivation Tracker

	Completed ✔
Fast Break Goal 1:	
Fast Break Goal 2:	
Fast Break Goal 3:	
Motivation Strategy 1:	
Motivation Strategy 2:	
Motivation Strategy 3:	

SparkTime
CHALLENGES AND ACCOMPLISHMENTS

JOIN US ONLINE

As a free bonus provided only to people who've purchased this book, we have built a section of the SparkPeople Website that contains exclusive bonus material just for readers. You will see me and other SparkPeople experts and members interacting here. This bonus material includes:

- An automatic SparkPoints tracker you can use to log your SparkPoints from the book and be eligible for fun prizes

- Downloadable and interactive versions of some of the trackers found in this book

- Teams of other members from around the world reading the book

- Interactive recipe wheels that let you create your own 300- and 400-calorie recipes, and additional sample meal plans at 1200, 1500, and 1800 calories

- A connection to all the other great free features on SparkPeople.com, such as the nutrition and fitness trackers, daily updated content, e-mail newsletters, and support from millions of other members

- News about author events, member events, author blogs, and more from the SparkPeople experts and coaches

When you are finished with the book program, you'll be able to go online to continue reaching your goals. This information is found at SparkPeople.com/TheSpark. Put in this code on the site to access this exclusive bonus content: SPARKTIME.

ACKNOWLEDGMENTS

It's fun to write the acknowledgments for *The Spark* because our big idea for this book is to show how a small team of people are working together to spark a grassroots movement that truly has the potential to help tens of millions of people reach their goals.

This may have started with me and my story, but the spark then grew to include a passionate team of employees and now millions of members. Now I'm just a small part of something special. I joke that there's a reason the company isn't named ChrisPeople.com. It's all about a great team.

Here's my chance to thank everyone involved. Thanks to:

Tami Corwin for leading this entire book project. As a legend in this book category and a great person to work with, Tami was able to help us translate the magic happening on SparkPeople into book form. She also helped significantly with the writing and direction, keeping me sane and calm along the way.

Lynn Lauber for leading the writing of the book. Lynn has been wonderful to work with. She has a gift for bringing stories to life. We knew we needed someone special like Lynn to help tell this story.

Dave Heilmann and Josh Knepfle, the SparkPeople COO and CTO, respectively—in addition to my longtime friends. I've now worked with Dave and Josh for over a decade. Without their leadership, SparkPeople wouldn't exist today.

The SparkPeople nutrition, fitness, and motivation coaches passionate about sharing their expertise to help people. Coach Nicole Nichols, Coach Dean Anderson, and Coach Becky Hand all helped tremendously with the book. Special thanks to Coach "One Take" Nicole for starring in the companion exercise DVD.

Other SparkPeople team members who directly helped with the book: Kelly Berger, Beth Cavanaugh, Grant Miller, Stepfanie Romine, and Jenny Uhlmansiek.

The entire SparkPeople team. This team works harder and smarter than any team I've ever been on. They continually add new features and content to help people. It's not easy for 25 people to handle a complex Website that receives more than 10 million visits per month, but they make it look easy. Here are all the team members not already mentioned: Dominic Acito, Kevin Carroll, Catherine Cram, Samantha Donohue, Paul Elfers,

Cougs Firsich, Brian Franklin, Elliott Giles, Angie Heilmann, Nancy Howard, Tanya Jollife, Tom Kennedy, Julie Knepfle, Jeremy Martin, Sean McCosh, Tim Metzner, Denise Tausig (with help from husband, Matt), and Rachel Von Nida.

Every SparkPeople member working hard to reach goals and spread the spark to friends, family, and co-workers. Thanks to you this has turned into a grassroots movement spreading around the world.

The Hay House team led by Reid Tracy. Hay House is an amazing partner we'd recommend to any author. Other members of the Hay House team include Anne Barthel, Tricia Breidenthal, Jacqui Clark, Laura Koch, Jeannie Liberati, Sally Mason, Charles McStravick, Margarete Nielsen, and John Thompson.

Patty Gift, our Hay House Editor. Patty helped push us at a crucial point to get this right.

Stephanie Tade, our agent. Stephanie helped us believe early on this could be a big, important book.

Early SparkPeople member Cyprinodon. She helped bring the online community to life.

Pat Searle, my co-worker at Procter & Gamble. My interaction with Pat was the "spark" that eventually led to the creation of SparkPeople.

Rob Ratterman, Tom Duvall, and Wally Carroll, my partners at Up4Sale.com. Without the success of Up4Sale.com, I wouldn't have been able to start SparkPeople. I also learned a great deal from Rob that I still use today.

Jeff Skoll and Pierre Omidyar, the first President and Founder of eBay, respectively. Jeff and Pierre are great models for for-profit social entrepreneurship leaders.

Steve Case, Co-Founder of AOL and Founder of Revolution. Steve is the only outside investor in SparkPeople and is passionate about improving healthcare.

John Pepper, Chairman of the Board at Disney. John was an incredible early role model when I was at Procter & Gamble. John motivated me to try my best to lead the right way.

Joe Downie, my brother. Joe helped put together and test important parts of the SparkPeople program.

Joe Hale, a longtime SparkPeople Board member, who is passionate about the Spark-People mission.

General Colin Powell, for paying me possibly the best compliment of my life. His response when I told him that I believe SparkPeople can change the course of American history by helping us reach our full potential still motivates me today. His encouragement inspires my hard work in pursuit of this goal.

My Mom, for showing me the value of hard work and persevering to reach goals.

My wife, Karina, and my two boys for being with me every step of the way on this grand adventure! My two boys are my greatest motivators to stay healthy so I can keep up with them and help them lead the next generation of SparkPeople.

ENDNOTES

Chapter 2: CORNERSTONE: Focus

1. Charles Garfield, *Peak Performers* (New York: William Morrow, 1986), 31.

2. Scott Adams, *The Dilbert Future: Thriving on Business Stupidity in the 21st Century* (New York: HarperBusiness, 1998), 250.

3. Viktor Frankl, *Man's Search for Meaning* (Boston: Beacon Press, 2006), 75.

Chapter 3: CORNERSTONE: Fitness

1. American Institute of Stress, http://www.stress.org/americas.htm.

2. T. G. Allison, D. E. Williams, et al., "Medical and Economic Costs of Psychologic Distress in Patients with Coronary Artery Disease," *Mayo Clinic Proceedings* 70, no. 8 (1995): 734–742.

3. U.S. National Highway Traffic Safety Administration, http://www.nhtsa.dot.gov /cars/rules/rulings/priorityplan/

Chapter 4: CORNERSTONE: Fire

1. Brian Dakss, "Reeve Tributes Keep Pouring In," October 12, 2004, http://www.cbsnews.com/stories/2004/10/12/earlyshow/health/health_ news/main648782.shtml

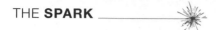

2.   Alice Park, "What's Driving Dara Torres," *Time,* August 4, 2008, http://www.time.com/time/specials/packages/article/0,28804,1819129_1819134_1825304,00.html

Chapter 5: CORNERSTONE: Positive Force

1.   John Pepper, *What Really Matters: Service, Leadership, People, and Values* (New Haven: Yale University Press, 2007), 268.

2.   Kevin Cullen, "A Head with a Heart," *The Boston Globe,* March 12, 2009.

3.   Martin Seligman, *Authentic Happiness: Using the New Positive Psychology to Realize Your Potential for Lasting Fulfillment* (New York: Free Press, 2004), 53.

4.   Johns Hopkins University, "Gaining Health While Giving Back to the Community," April 6, 2004, http://www.hopkinsmedicine.org/Press_releases/2004/04_06_04.html.

Chapter 7: Healthy Diet Habits

1.   Institute of Medicine of the National Academies, http://www.iom.edu/?id=4340&redirect=0

2.   University of Chicago Medical Center, "Sleep Loss Boosts Appetite, May Encourage Weight Gain," *ScienceDaily*, December 7, 2004, http://www.sciencedaily.com/releases/2004/12/041206210355.htm.

3.   Helen Pearson, "Medicine: Sleep It Off," *Nature,* September 21, 2006: 261–263.

Chapter 8: Lifestyle Change

1.   Nicholas A. Christakis, M.D., Ph.D., M.P.H., and James H. Fowler, Ph.D., "The Spread of Obesity in a Large Social Network over 32 Years," *New England Journal of Medicine* 357, no. 4 (2007): 1866–1868.

2. Amy Paturel, "The ABC's of Slim," *Women's Health,* January, February, 2008, http://www.womenshealthmag.com/weight-loss/weight-loss-secrets.

Chapter 9: Spread the Spark

1. Susan Lark, M.D.,"Susan Lark, MD Says 'Volunteer' Your Way to Good Health this Holiday Season," NewsGuide.us, October 31, 2008, http://www.newsguide.us/health-medical/mental-health/Susan-Lark-MD-Says-Volunteer-Your-Way-to-Good-Health-this-Holiday-Season/.

2. Allan Luks, *The Healing Power of Doing Good* (New York: iUniverse, 2001).

ABOUT THE AUTHOR

Chris Downie, commonly known as "SparkGuy," is the founder and CEO of Spark-People, Inc., an online initiative aimed at helping people achieve their personal goals to live happier, healthier lifestyles.

As he developed the program, Chris was motivated to leave his position at Procter & Gamble to cofound an online auction company named Up4Sale. Up4Sale grew into the second-largest person-to-person online auction site and was eventually acquired by eBay in 1998. This entrepreneurial success story inspired Chris to give back to others through his brainchild, SparkPeople.

With his business acumen and strong sense of philanthropic duty, Chris and his team have led SparkPeople to become the most active diet and fitness Website in the U.S., according to comScore, Inc., garnering the attention of media outlets including *The New York Times*, ABC News, FOX TV, the *Today* show, and many more.

As SparkPeople's motivation expert, Chris corresponds directly with members every day. Since 2000, he has written countless letters celebrating members' victories and offering encouraging words at times of struggle.

Website: **www.SparkPeople.com**

HAY HOUSE TITLES OF RELATED INTEREST

YOU CAN HEAL YOUR LIFE, the movie, starring Louise L. Hay & Friends
(available as a 1-DVD program and an expanded 2-DVD set)
Watch the trailer at: **www.LouiseHayMovie.com**

THE SHIFT, the movie,
starring Dr. Wayne W. Dyer
(available as a 1-DVD program and an expanded 2-DVD set)
Watch the trailer at: **www.DyerMovie.com**

✻

BE HAPPY: Release the Power of Happiness in YOU,
by Robert Holden, Ph.D.

*THE CORE BALANCE DIET: 4 Weeks to Boost Your Metabolism and
Lose Weight for Good,* by Marcelle Pick

*EXCUSES BEGONE!: How to Change Lifelong, Self-Defeating
Thinking Habits,* by Dr. Wayne W. Dyer

*LIGHTEN UP!: The Authentic and Fun Way to Lose Your
Weight and Your Worries,* by Loretta LaRoche

PLAYGROUND PUMP: The Workout, by Chris L. Rauchnot

*RECIPES FOR HEALTH BLISS: Using NatureFoods & Lifestyle Choices to
Rejuvenate Your Body & Life,* by Susan Smith Jones, Ph.D.

All of the above are available at your local bookstore,
or may be ordered by contacting Hay House.

We hope you enjoyed this Hay House book. If you'd like
to receive our online catalog featuring additional information
on Hay House books and products, or if you'd like to find
out more about the Hay Foundation, please contact:

Hay House, Inc., P.O. Box 5100, Carlsbad, CA 92018-5100

(760) 431-7695 or **(800) 654-5126**
(760) 431-6948 (fax) or **(800) 650-5115 (fax)**
www.hayhouse.com® • **www.hayfoundation.org**

✳

Published and distributed in Australia by: Hay House Australia Pty. Ltd.,
18/36 Ralph St., Alexandria NSW 2015 • *Phone:* 612-9669-4299
Fax: 612-9669-4144 • www.hayhouse.com.au

Published and distributed in the United Kingdom by: Hay House UK, Ltd.,
292B Kensal Rd., London W10 5BE • *Phone:* 44-20-8962-1230
Fax: 44-20-8962-1239 • www.hayhouse.co.uk

Published and distributed in the Republic of South Africa by:
Hay House SA (Pty), Ltd., P.O. Box 990, Witkoppen 2068
Phone/Fax: 27-11-467-8904 • info@hayhouse.co.za • www.hayhouse.co.za

Published in India by: Hay House Publishers India,
Muskaan Complex, Plot No. 3, B-2, Vasant Kunj, New Delhi 110 070
Phone: 91-11-4176-1620 • *Fax:* 91-11-4176-1630 • www.hayhouse.co.in

Distributed in Canada by: Raincoast, 9050 Shaughnessy St., Vancouver, B.C. V6P 6E5
Phone: (604) 323-7100 • *Fax:* (604) 323-2600 • www.raincoast.com

✳

<u>Take Your Soul on a Vacation</u>

Visit **www.HealYourLife.com**® to regroup, recharge, and reconnect
with your own magnificence. Featuring blogs, mind-body-spirit
news, and life-changing wisdom from Louise Hay and friends.

Visit **www.HealYourLife.com** today!

Mind Your Body,
Mend Your Spirit

Hay House is the ultimate resource for inspirational and health-conscious books, audio programs, movies, events, e-newsletters, member communities, and much more.

Visit **www.hayhouse.com®** today and nourish your soul.

UPLIFTING EVENTS

Join your favorite authors at live events in a city near you or log on to **www.hayhouse.com** to visit with Hay House authors online during live, interactive Web events.

INSPIRATIONAL RADIO

Daily inspiration while you're at work or at home. Enjoy radio programs featuring your favorite authors, streaming live on the Internet 24/7 at **HayHouseRadio.com®**. Tune in and tune up your spirit!

VIP STATUS

Join the Hay House VIP membership program today and enjoy exclusive discounts on books, CDs, calendars, card decks, and more. You'll also receive 10% off all event reservations (excluding cruises). Visit **www.hayhouse.com/wisdom** to join the Hay House Wisdom Community™.

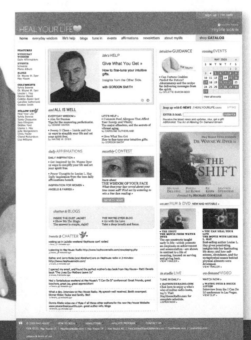